Don't bite off more than you can chew.
Successful weight loss is achieved
one small change at a time.

The Small Change Diet is based on ten key steps that will help you turn your bad habits into good ones and give you immediate weight loss results and a lifetime of health:

1. Create a healthy eating schedule.

2. Eat more fruits and vegetables.

3. Cut empty beverage calories.

4. Increase fiber intake.

5. Reduce the undercover calories of dressings and sauces.

6. Eat leaner meats.

7. Find the right fats and lose the bad fats.

8. Curb sugar and salt cravings.

9. Stay healthy in social situations.

10. Exercise.

**The Small Change Diet is also available
as an eBook.**

What are Registered Dietitians saying about Keri Gans and *The Small Change Diet* on Amazon?

"**211 pages of tips, tricks, and advice from a real pro**. . . . Keri cuts through the clutter and gives you back-to-the-basics advice that is realistic and doable. One of my favorite parts of the book is the Questions & Answers (called "Small Change Solutions") throughout each chapter because they offer **sensible strategies to real-life scenarios, tricky situations, common challenges, and dieting excuses. This book is a winner!**"

—Dawn Jackson Blatner, RD, author of
The Flexitarian Diet

"**This is definitely a book that I will recommend to all my patients.** It puts into words what I try to convey in our sessions. This is **an excellent resource** for all practitioners and great for anyone who is looking to make changes in an approachable way. Thank you, Ms. Gans, for giving us **a sound, sensible approach to an overwhelming issue!**"

—J. Elizabeth Smythe, RD, CDN, CPT,
Media Representative, The New York State
Dietetic Association

"As a registered dietitian, author, and mother of two, and an advocate for making small, realistic, sensible, and practical changes to improve eating, fitness, and health habits, **I highly recommend *The Small Change Diet*.** . . . After reading this book, **you'll likely eat more healthfully, and enjoy the many physical and mental benefits of a more balanced diet**."

—Elisa Zied, MS, RD, CDN, author of
Nutrition at Your Fingertips

More praise for *The Small Change Diet*

"A smart, totally manageable way to tackle weight loss. With Keri's expert guidance, you'll train yourself to gradually give up unhealthy eating habits and replace them with slimming strategies proven to shed pounds and boost energy!"

—Joy Bauer, MS, RD, nutrition expert for
the *Today* Show

"Small changes can make huge differences. Keri gives super-practical, easy-to-digest advice that anyone can benefit from!"

—Lisa Lillien, #1 *New York Times* bestselling author of
the Hungry Girl series

"The newest diet book on the market is one of the smartest ones ever written."

—Tara Gidus, MS, RD, CSSD, LD/N, author of
Pregnancy Cooking & Nutrition for Dummies,
Healthline

"Keri addresses our quick-fix culture head-on. . . . Start reading any chapter, and you will find a smart and sensible strategy on how to tackle the problem standing between you, a healthy weight, and a balanced food and drink intake."

—Kristin Voorhees, Healthcare Relations Manager,
National Foundation for Celiac Awareness (NFCA)

"Gans keeps her solutions manageable by grounding them in real life."

—Elizabeth Willse, Women's Voices for Change

"A refreshing and practical guide. . . . A terrific resource."

—Sandra Frank, EdD, RD, LDN,
Dietitians Online Blog

The Small Change Diet

▼▲▼▲▼▲▼▲▼▲▼

10 Steps to a Thinner, Healthier You

▼▲▼▲▼▲▼▲▼▲▼

Keri Gans,

MS, RD, CDN

POCKET BOOKS

NEW YORK LONDON TORONTO SYDNEY NEW DELHI

Pocket Books
A Division of Simon & Schuster, Inc.
1230 Avenue of the Americas
New York, NY 10020

This publication contains the opinions and ideas of the author. It is sold with the understanding that the author and publisher are not engaged in rendering health services in the book. The reader should consult his or her own medical and health providers as appropriate before adopting any of the suggestions in this book or drawing inferences from it.

The author and publisher specifically disclaim all responsibility for any liability, loss, or risk, personal or otherwise, which is incurred as a consequence, directly or indirectly, of the use and application of any of the contents of this book.

First Pocket Books paperback edition January 2012

POCKET and colophon are registered trademarks of Simon & Schuster, Inc.

For information about special discounts for bulk purchases, please contact Simon & Schuster Special Sales at 1-866-506-1949 or business@simonandschuster.com.

The Simon & Schuster Speakers Bureau can bring authors to your live event. For more information or to book an event, contact the Simon & Schuster Speakers Bureau at 1-866-248-3049 or visit our website at www.simonspeakers.com.

Cover design by Mary Ann Smith.
Cover photography: fries © Getty Images; tape measure © superstock.

Manufactured in the United States of America

10 9 8 7 6 5 4 3 2

ISBN: 978-1-4516-0890-8
ISBN: 978-1-4516-0893-9 (ebook)

CONTENTS

▼▲▼▲▼▲▼▲▼

The
Small Change
Diet

INTRODUCTION
▽▲▽▲▽▲▽▲▽

We live in a fast-paced world of express lanes and overnight delivery. To get ahead, we juggle work and family and often tackle more than we can handle. No pain, no gain, we preach. We are conditioned to believe that faster is better and that the more you do and the harder you work, the more successful you are. As a result, most people imagine the only way to lose weight is to do something drastic and severe. They spend way too much time counting calories, restricting their food choices, and eliminating entire food groups. They create too many unrealistic food rules for themselves, and they're miserable. At the end of the day, they find themselves discouraged when the pounds don't drop off fast enough or they gain back all the weight. Some people become so disappointed that they stop trying altogether. Sound familiar?

It sure sounds familiar to me. As a registered dietitian with a private practice in Manhattan, I see this folly all the time in my clients. They sincerely want to lose weight, but they've been on so many fad or crash diets that they've lost sight of a very important truth: To lose weight, you must eat *normally*. With portion size, and health, in mind. I help them accomplish this by retraining their habits, so they can form new habits that have a decisive impact on their weight. The cornerstone of my belief: The changes that will make the most impact are often the smallest ones, including, Don't be in a hurry.

The real truth is if you take on too much and lose weight too quickly, you will gain it all back, and then some. Why doesn't quick weight loss stick? Because when it happens too fast, it means you didn't train yourself to change bad habits for the long haul, and without these long-term changes, eventually you are right back where you started. Many of my patients continued to make this same grueling, quick-fix mistake until they came to see me. I taught them to slow down and focus on ten key changes—the Small Change Diet that I am about to share with you—that finally gave them the weight loss success that lasts a lifetime. I've worked with hundreds of clients who have lost an average of ten to sixty pounds, and they have all kept it off for years. So can you.

Weight loss doesn't have to feel like another race to the finish line, another unrealistic pressure you have to manage. Whether you are trying to shed ten pounds or a hundred, it didn't take you days to gain that unwanted weight. It took months, probably years, of not-so-great habits—like skipping meals, reaching for fried food, sipping sugary beverages—to pack on the pounds. Why should anyone, including you, expect to lose the weight overnight? I'm here to tell you that consistency wins the race. Relax. Take a breath. Don't bite off more than you can chew. Healthy weight loss is achieved one change at a time.

Don't get me wrong; all of my patients also lose weight immediately, and so will you. For instance, most people lose five to ten pounds with each incorporated change over several weeks, depending on their lifestyle and weight. Stop drinking soda every day: Drop five pounds. Start eating breakfast: Drop another five pounds. Eat fish once a week: *bam*, another two pounds. Each change delivers its own instant results depending on your lifestyle and needs.

The big difference between my plan and so-called quick fixes is that the Small Change Diet doesn't require you to be perfect from day one. It's about really training yourself to do one healthy change before expecting yourself to tackle another. It's turning smart habits into second nature. And best of all, by making one change at a time, you don't feel deprived as you lose the weight. I always ask my patients the same question: "Do you feel like you are on a diet?" The answer is almost always no—make that, "No!" The Small Change Diet gives you permission and the tools to adopt a healthier eating regime, one Small Change at a time. Are you with me? Then let's go!

The Small Change Diet is based on the following ten key changes that will help you turn your bad habits into good ones and give you immediate weight loss results and a lifetime of health:

1. Create a healthy eating schedule.

2. Brighten your plate, naturally.

3. Think before you drink (sip, guzzle, or chug).

4. Give your carbs a makeover.

5. Go easy on the "extras" and make savory swaps for old standbys.

6. Skinny your meat.

7. Eat the right kinds (and amounts) of fat.

8. Tame your sweet tooth and your saltshaker.

9. Share food and good times with advance planning—and without guilt.

10. Get moving.

The book is organized around ten key Small Changes, each providing a progressive Small Change Plan for you to master and reap its instant rewards. Once you train yourself to adopt one change, you move on to another. *You* decide which changes to focus on and when it is time to make another. Once you've made all ten Small Changes, you will not only achieve an entirely healthier, thinner you, but you will also be able to easily maintain your weight loss for good.

If you have a basic understanding of good nutrition, none of the ten key changes are shockingly new. The hard part is putting them into practice, which can seem overwhelming. (Give up *soda*? Eat breakfast *every day*?!) Relax. On this plan, you'll learn how to tackle each "overwhelming" change by breaking it down into small, doable steps that reward you on many levels—better health, continued and sustainable weight loss, and new, tastier flavors.

HAVE A REASON AND A GOAL

Before we begin, you must decide *why* you are changing. Losing weight isn't easy, but it's easier to rise to the challenge if you can see, very clearly, why you want to reach your goals. For some, it is the fear of illness or the desire to stop preventable diseases—like heart disease—where excessive weight is a risk factor; perhaps diabetes or high cholesterol runs in your family and you don't want that to be your fate. Maybe you want to feel better and fit into that favorite pair of jeans again. Or perhaps you're simply not happy with how you look anymore. Find a reason that is really going to motivate you.

Once you have a reason, set your weight loss goal. How many pounds do you want to lose, and by when? In my experience, this is where most people get overzealous. Be realistic, and set a goal that you can meet. Healthy weight loss should be gradual, one to two pounds per week. One to two pounds may not sound like much to you now, but think of it this way: Every pound you lose is also a pound you don't gain. A pound a week is ten pounds in ten weeks. Over the course of a year, you could lose fifty to one hundred pounds. Stop setting yourself up for failure, and you will find out how easy it is to succeed.

HOW TO USE THE BOOK

Each chapter introduces a core Small Change and then offers a Small Change Plan that breaks the change into even smaller steps to take over the course of each week (or weeks). There is no true time limit. You can take as long as you need to make a Small Change. But for this to work, you must complete one change before moving on to another. For example, the first Small Change Plan is for creating a healthy eating schedule and looks like this:

Your Small Change Plan

1. Eat breakfast.

2. Eat lunch.

3. Eat every three to four hours.

4. Eat dinner.

5. Get at least seven hours of sleep.

The weight loss and pace is 100 percent tailored to you and your body. How much weight you lose and how long it takes you to master the change will vary according to your own strengths and lifestyle. For instance, you might find that it takes you longer to curb your cravings than it takes you to up your fiber. You could potentially take on one Small Change per week, or it could take you two or more weeks for each change—and that's okay. In fact, rushing through any of these changes actually can be counterproductive. So give yourself a week of successful follow-through—minimum—for each one. The ultimate goal isn't to swiftly check off the list, but to ensure that you can stick to your new, healthy habits.

Each chapter ends with a Small Change Success Test that will help you assess whether you have mastered your Small Change and are ready to move on. Whether you've lost five pounds or dropped a dress size, don't take on a new change until you pass the Success Test. Then, and only then, will you enjoy weight loss that lasts.

MEASURE YOUR SUCCESS

One of the best ways to keep yourself honest and accountable during your quest for change is to record your progress, including what you are eating. When I first started my private practice, I used to hate to ask people to keep track of what they were putting into their mouths. I thought it was unreasonable and impractical. After all, who wants to write down everything they are eating every day? *How annoying,* I thought. But after ten years of counseling patients for weight loss, I have totally changed my mind about this. Keeping a food journal helps immensely, and I have seen far more success from patients who record than those who don't. Food journals create accountability and provide an instant overview of how you are doing. I urge you to use this powerful tool.

I suggest one of three ways for food journaling:

1. Buy a small notebook that can fit into your purse or briefcase.

2. Create a template on your computer that you can easily access.

3. Buy an application for your smartphone or PDA.

Find a way to journal that fits your lifestyle. Record every meal you have throughout the day and the quantities, including beverages, snacks, and even "nibbles" (like that handful of pretzels or M&M's). The time of day that you eat your meals and snacks is also very important, as you will see in the following chapters, so make sure to note that, as well. In addition, record your daily exercises, whether that means going to the gym, doing yoga, or just taking a long walk.

If you use your weight as a tool to measure your success, weigh yourself on the same day of the week, at the same time of day. Consistency is important if you want a true reading. You will drive yourself crazy if you weigh every day because factors like salt consumption can make the scale jump up and down. If the scale didn't move since the week before, review your food journal to see in black and white how successful you have been on following your Small Change Plan. For example, if you were on Small Change 2 and you see from your journal that you added fruits and vegetables to your plate on only three out of seven nights, then you know you still have work to do on making this change. It is very important not to get discouraged, even if the scale isn't moving as quickly as you'd like it to. Use *all* results, whether positive or negative, as an opportunity to measure your success.

If the scale is not the tool for you, go ahead and use the fit test. Hey, we all know when our pants are too tight, the zipper won't go up, the shirt doesn't button, etc. You don't need a scale to tell you the news. Use your clothes as your guide. Like the scale, they don't lie. For those of you who get needlessly obsessed with the numbers (weighing yourself every day and then some), consider passing on the "weigh-in" and opt for a "try on."

So are you ready? Are you committed to change, one step at a time?

Are you set? Have you determined your reasons and your goal?

Then go! No deprivation, no struggles. Just ten Small Changes that will make a *big* difference.

SMALL CHANGE 1

▼▲▼▲▼▲▼▲▼

Create a Healthy Eating Schedule

It may sound counterintuitive but many people have difficulty losing weight because they skip meals throughout the day. If you skip meals, you *will* be hungrier the next time you eat, and you *will* overeat. Contrary to popular belief, overeating often stems from not eating enough of the right foods at the right time. Study after study shows that you will consume more calories at the end of the day when you skip meals and snacks.

Be honest: Are you a meal skipper? Are you starved at lunch or dinner because you didn't eat enough earlier in the day? Do you tend to eat sporadically but are never really satisfied? If you can answer yes to any of these questions, you do not have a healthy eating schedule. In this chapter, you don't need to focus on what you are eating but rather *when* you are eating. Of course, I'll still offer you some smart food choices, but we'll tackle *what* you're eating in more detail in later chapters.

For some, meal skipping isn't deliberate; it simply happens on a daily basis because of lifestyle. Others skip meals on purpose because they think they're eliminating calories. I've heard all the excuses. Most of my patients used to skip breakfast because they weren't hungry. Lunch? Not when they had that afternoon meeting to get ready for. And dinner? Maybe they opted for bar snacks or didn't have time to eat lunch until 4:00 p.m. and felt full come dinnertime. No matter how busy or tired you are, you should *never, ever* skip meals. One of the most important steps toward losing weight is to eat regularly.

WHAT DOES A HEALTHY EATING SCHEDULE LOOK LIKE?

You should begin your day with an early breakfast, followed by a well-chosen lunch and a satisfying dinner, with two to three well-timed snacks. Aim to eat every three to four hours, and never go more than five hours without eating. The Small Change Meal Wheel on page 15 shows you a healthy eating schedule. Each slice of the wheel represents the three-hour time period in which you should eat. The example is based on a 6 a.m. wake-up time. Plug in your own wake-up time and adjust the subsequent times for a personalized Meal Wheel.

The Small Change Meal Wheel

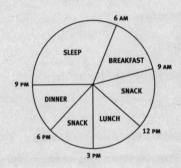

Don't jump into reforming your whole routine at once and struggling through a "perfect day" or a series of perfect days. Trying to tackle too much can lead to failure. Instead, follow the clock and start with the first meal of the day. Once you feel comfortable with breakfast, move on to lunch. Once lunch feels like part of your normal routine, start changing your dinner. When you can manage three meals a day, move on to snacks, and then finally your sleeping schedule.

Keep your food journal up to date, recording every meal and snack that you eat over the next two weeks. This way you can better monitor your meal schedule. Before you know it, your healthy routine will feel as comfortable as sliding into your favorite pair of jeans.

Your Small Change Plan

1. Eat breakfast.

2. Eat lunch.

3. Eat every three to four hours.

4. Eat dinner.

5. Get at least seven hours of sleep.

LET'S START AT THE BEGINNING . . .
WITH BREAKFAST!

If you want to be thin, you need to start doing what thin people do, and that is *eat breakfast*. Want to lose fifteen pounds? Instead of signing up for a trendy 6 a.m. gym class, you're better off signing up for breakfast. When Stephanie, twenty-four, first came to me, she was skipping breakfast and consuming too many calories later in the day. After two weeks of simply committing to breakfast, Stephanie lost three pounds. "I feel fuller now during the day," she said. Thirteen months later and still thirty pounds lighter, Stephanie continues to enjoy her nonfat plain yogurt, blueberries, and high-fiber cereal in the morning.

After being in private practice for more than ten years, I have heard every possible excuse for skipping breakfast:

I have no time to eat breakfast in the morning.

Small Change Solution: Breakfast can be very quick and simple. It does not require a lot of effort to prepare or cost a lot of money. Do you have five minutes for a bathroom break? Or one extra "snooze" when your alarm clock goes off? Then you have time for breakfast. Five minutes is all it really has to take. You can eat breakfast at home, in your office, or even on the run.

I am not hungry in the morning.

Small Change Solution: In my practice, I have seen many breakfast dodgers who can't remember the last time their breakfast was more than a cup of coffee. By lunchtime, they are *way* hungrier than they should be and wind up making poor meal decisions. Once you start eating breakfast regularly, you will find that your appetite changes in the morning. You will be hungry when you wake up, and better yet, your lunch choices will improve.

I don't want to waste the calories.

Small Change Solution: When I hear a patient complain about "wasting calories" by eating breakfast, I just shake my head—nothing could be further from the truth. Breakfast is not only an opportunity to kick-start your metabolism and your day, it is also proven that eating breakfast leads you to eat fewer calories throughout the day.

How many hours are you up before eating breakfast? Ideally, I suggest eating within one to two hours of waking up. Typically the longer you wait to eat, the hungrier you will be. If you cannot imagine eating breakfast, start off slowly. Grab an energy bar, a piece of fruit, or a slice of toast. You can eat it at home, on the way to work or school, or at your desk. The goal is to incorporate breakfast into your day, every day. It might not be 100 percent ideal at the beginning, but that's where the Small Change solutions will move you along. Your first goal is to make breakfast as natural for you as brushing your teeth in the morning.

To keep it interesting, here's a shopping list of must-have breakfast items to stock in your kitchen. You can find these items anywhere, and three favorites are usually enough to satisfy dieters:

- Oatmeal
- High-fiber cold cereal
- Nonfat or low-fat milk
- Nonfat or low-fat yogurt
- Nonfat or low-fat cottage cheese
- Eggs/Egg whites
- Natural peanut butter or other nut butters
- Whole-wheat English muffin
- Fruit
- Crushed walnuts or almonds

MAKE BREAKFAST—AND THEN MAKE IT BETTER!

Once you get used to eating something, anything, in the morning, it's time to graduate to healthier breakfast options that will undoubtedly prove more satisfying. But before you go any further, stop and congratulate yourself on eating breakfast . . . no small feat if this is a new habit for you, and it doesn't go unnoticed by your body.

A good way to gauge whether your breakfast is balanced is to take note of how long it takes before you feel hungry again. If you feel hungry an hour later, usually it is because your breakfast was too high in carbohydrates, loaded with sugar, and/or not high enough in fiber and protein. Many of my patients must be weaned off of their early-morning, low-fiber choices, such as buttered rolls, low-fiber cereals, bagels and cream cheese, croissants, and doughnuts. The more fiber your breakfast contains, the longer it takes to digest, causing you to feel fuller longer. Sometimes you might find yourself too hungry because you eliminated fat. Shocking, I know. The ultimate goal with breakfast is to have a well-balanced meal with high-fiber carbohydrates, some lean protein, and a little healthy fat. (As you'll see, this balance is important in lunch, dinner, and snacks, as well.) We'll explore lean proteins and healthy fats in more detail in later chapters. For now, here are some easy Small Change Breakfast Tips to help balance your breakfast:

Small Change Breakfast Tips

1. Make oatmeal with milk (non- or low-fat) for more protein.

2. Add cinnamon to oats for sweetness instead of sugar.

3. If a bowl of cereal leaves you hungry, add 1 hard-boiled egg on the side for additional protein.

4. Make scrambled eggs with 1 whole egg and 2 or 3 egg whites.

5. Top cereal or yogurt with nuts if choosing nonfat milk/yogurt. The added fat will help you feel more satiated.

6. To lightly sweeten plain yogurt, add 1 teaspoon of jam or whole fruit.

7. Choose a piece of whole fruit instead of juice. Juice adds calories without the benefit of fiber.

8. If you can't pass on your bagel in the morning, scoop out the inside.

9. Try "buttering" your bread with 100 percent vegetable oil spread instead of butter. If you're not ready to part with butter, switch to more spreadable whipped butter instead of sticks, and you'll consume less saturated fat.

10. Switch from regular cream cheese to low-fat cream cheese.

DON'T BE OUT TO LUNCH WHEN IT COMES TO LUNCH

As your healthy eating routine develops, lunch must become an integral part of your day. It fuels all your activities for the afternoon and sets your eating rhythm until dinner. If you make poor decisions at lunch, most likely you will continue to make them until you go to bed.

The workweek is especially hard. Most of my patients are so busy at their jobs that they don't make time to eat lunch. Or they find it hard to eat healthfully in the office when colleagues are picking up fast food for everyone. Some of them work from home and nibble all day, never sitting down to a real meal. On weekends, many people run around all afternoon and skip their lunch break, which sets them up to overeat when they finally sit down for dinner.

Also, the longer you wait in between breakfast and lunch, the hungrier you will be. The goal is to eat lunch four to five hours after breakfast. If breakfast is at 8 a.m. and lunch is at noon, you are all set. Depending on where you work (or if you are in school), you may have little control over when lunch is scheduled. If breakfast is at 7 a.m. and lunch doesn't happen until 1 p.m., the gap is too long. Later, we will address how to use snacks to mind the gap.

Besides the issue of timing, there are other lunch issues I've seen my clients struggle with.

I am too busy at work to think about lunch.

Small Change Solution: Brown-bagging your lunch allows you to move your lunch prep to the time of day that is easiest for you. You can make your lunch the evening before you go to bed, the morning before work, or after work when you get home. When you bring your lunch, you don't have to think about it, you just have to eat it. And if you are going to be stuck in a meeting, eat half of it before going in and the other half when you get out.

I deliberately skip lunch because I want to save calories for dinner.

Small Change Solution: Talk about penny-wise and pound-foolish! Don't skip lunch, even if you think breakfast was excessive or you plan on a big dinner. Eat something light. Don't let a morning slip-up or an evening indulgence change what you should be doing in the afternoon. Two wrongs don't make a right. The calories you "save" at lunch will be doubled later.

I nibble all day and before I know it the day is over and I never sat down to an actual meal.

Small Change Solution: It's hard to get all of the right nutrients that will fuel your body and keep you feeling full when you are constantly munching. Stick to your meal schedule and pay attention to the times you should eat lunch and snacks. Don't enter the kitchen for food unless it is a scheduled snack or meal time.

LUNCH MAKEOVERS THAT WON'T LEAVE YOU STARVING (OR SLEEPY)

At lunch, we usually overdo the fat. The most effective way to stay on track until dinner is to have a balance of fiber, lean protein, and healthy fats. Do not eliminate any one food group. If your lunch is filled with fatty foods like French fries, BLTs, or cheeseburgers, you will feel sluggish. If you eat huge portions of carbs such as pasta, you'll feel a boost that will wear off quickly. If you don't include enough lean protein, such as tuna, tofu, chicken, or healthy fat (i.e., nuts, seeds, avocado), you'll be hungry an hour later. To feel energized and satisfied for three to four hours, try these Small Change Lunch Tips.

Small Change Lunch Tips

1. Have a piece of fruit for dessert. This helps fill you up and completes the meal.

2. Choose 2 slices of whole-wheat bread for your sandwich. Avoid rolls, heroes, or buns, which tend to have more calories and less fiber than sliced whole-grain breads.

3. Add protein (i.e., chicken, turkey, egg) to your tossed salad. Otherwise you will still feel hungry.

4. Don't turn a salad into a high-fat, high-calorie disaster. Avoid creamy dressings, as well as "extras" like bacon bits and oily croutons.

5. If you're still hungry, add a pickle to your meal.

6. Instead of chips or fries with your sandwich, choose vegetables or fruit.

7. Ask for dressings and sauces on the side.

8. Request light mayonnaise for your tuna salad, egg salad, or chicken salad.

9. Peruse restaurant buffets first without your
    plate, and then decide what you really want.

10. Build your sandwich with veggies, such as
    tomatoes, cucumber, lettuce, and onions, not
    high-fat cheeses, extra meats, or rich spreads.

A healthy lunch can either be purchased or you can
make it yourself and bring it to work. If brown-
bagging isn't for you, don't sweat it. Order food.
Eat with your colleagues. Eat at your desk. Just eat
lunch.

WHAT'S FOR DINNER?

If you have been following your new healthy eating
routine, you will be able to approach dinner with a
little more clarity. Most people don't skip dinner, but
they do skip it mentally. They eat whatever is available. Just like all your other meals, dinner needs to
be a balance of fiber, lean protein, and healthy fats.
The right balance prevents overeating or undereating. Overeating leads to excess calorie consumption,
but as discussed undereating can also do the same. If
you're unsatisfied after a poorly chosen dinner, you
will eat again before you go to bed and consume
more calories at the end of the day.

If you choose your dinner wisely, you're halfway there. But there are still a few dinnertime dilemmas that can steer you off course.

I work late and am too tired to cook, so I just eat snack foods. It's better than takeout, right?

Small Change Solution: Snacks are good, but they shouldn't replace meals. If you snack all night, you are never satisfied and end up consuming more calories than if you sat down for an actual meal. A home-cooked meal doesn't have to be labor intensive. A delicious healthy dinner can be created in very little time. For instance, broil a piece of fish, which takes only 15 minutes (or less, depending on thickness of fish), while you prepare whole-wheat couscous (about 5 minutes), and steam a veggie on the stove top or in the microwave (5 to 10 minutes, depending on cooking method). (See subsequent chapters for more cooking ideas.) Takeout doesn't have to be a diet disaster; just choose your selections wisely. Pick up a whole roasted chicken and eat one serving, which is approximately three ounces, skinless, preferably white meat. Choose roasted potatoes versus fried or mashed, and pick out a steamed or roasted veggie instead of sautéed or creamed.

I'm making dinner for my family or partner, and they claim they don't like healthy food.

Small Change Solution: You don't have to make different dinners for you and your family. Use the same basics for a healthy dinner on your family's favorites. For instance, grill the chicken instead of battering it for the chicken Parmesan. Put sauces on the side, so everyone can add the sauce to their own plates. And of course, be a health ringleader by substituting in healthier food options, like brown rice for white. You'll be surprised how many family members or partners will opt to eat more like you, and no one will feel deprived!

I enjoy going out for drinks with my friends and choose to drink my calories.

Small Change Solution: You should eat a meal *before* you go for drinks. If it is an early night, eat a snack. Without a meal or snack, you will most likely drink more and wind up eating poorly later. Calories from alcohol *do* count, and they don't give you the nutrients that keep you feeling satisfied.

PROTEIN IS GOOD—BUT BEWARE TOO MUCH OF A GOOD THING

At dinner, usually people eat too much protein. Think about your dinner plate. Is there room for lots of veggies? Or is your piece of meat or fish taking over more than its share?

Don't skimp on the veggies and whole grains (thinking the grains might add too many calories) and load up on the protein. An 8-ounce grilled chicken breast made with olive oil will provide around 480 calories, but if you did only 4 ounces of chicken with ½ cup brown rice, you would consume around 350 calories—and still have plenty of room for those veggies. These Small Change Dinner Tips below will help you turn your dinner don'ts into dinner dos:

Small Change Dinner Tips

1. If it looks like too much food, it is too much food.

2. Always start with a salad.

3. Ask for dressings and extras on the side.

4. Stay away from creamy sauces.

5. Don't eat bread with your dinner unless it is part of the sandwich.

6. The perfect dinner plate should be divided into three parts: ¼ of the plate should be high-fiber carbohydrates; ¼, lean protein; and ½, vegetables.

7. Roast, bake, steam, broil, and grill instead of sauté and fry.

8. Watch the alcohol. Liquid calories do count.

9. If you want seconds, have more veggies.

10. Eat fruit for dessert.

TOO LATE TO EAT?

It is never too late to eat dinner. Many people think that if they eat after 8 p.m. they will gain weight, but people who eat late at night gain weight only if they overeat. The longer you wait to eat any meal, the hungrier you will be, and if you ate lunch at 1 p.m. and don't eat dinner until 9 p.m., you are going to be starved! You will consume excess calories, which equals weight gain, plain and simple. Dinner should usually be three to four hours after your last snack.

✔ How's It Going?

Are you writing in your food journal every day? Are you recording all nibbles and beverages, including alcohol?

SNACK TIME!

Now that you are eating a healthy breakfast and lunch, you should feel hungry, not starving, three to four hours later. This means that your metabolism is working well and your small changes are making a difference already. A snack is an opportunity to continue fueling your body properly and to prevent you from making a disastrous food choice at lunchtime or dinner. I usually recommend that my patients include one snack between breakfast and lunch and one snack between lunch and dinner.

When Cybele, thirty-eight, first came to me, she had been trying for a while to lose weight without success. She even increased her exercise but the weight wasn't coming off. When I did a 24-hour dietary review, or 24-recall (the patient tells me everything that he ate for the last 24 hours), I discovered that she was having long gaps between her meals. As such, I encouraged her to include one snack per day. At her first follow-up two weeks later, Cybele felt like she was eating more, but she had actually lost four pounds. Eight months later, still fourteen pounds thinner, she is now eating two snacks a day.

If you had to choose only one snack per day, pick the one between lunch and dinner. I don't know anyone who doesn't complain about being hungry in the late afternoon or about being hungry when they get home from work. This snack is a *must* for everyone. If you happen to sleep late on the weekends, don't worry about having an a.m. snack. And if you happen not to be hungry after dinner, don't worry about having a p.m. snack. When you are eating after dinner, it usually has nothing to do with hunger—unless you are a night owl and stay up until 1–2 a.m. or it's 11 p.m. and you ate dinner at 6 p.m. Usually we eat out of boredom, habit, stress, or anxiety, but not true hunger.

Here's a shopping list of easy snacks to keep at home, in the office, or in your bag. You can find these items anywhere and usually three to five favorite choices are enough to satisfy anyone:

- String cheese or individual-size cheese
- Nonfat or low-fat yogurt or cottage cheese
- Hard-boiled egg
- Individual can of tuna
- Nuts (almonds, cashews, walnuts, pistachios, soy) or roasted edamame
- Whole-grain crisp bread or crackers
- Turkey slices

- Raw veggies

- Hummus

- Fruit

Now that you have a list of healthy foods to snack on, it's smooth sailing, right? Yes—just avoid the following trip-ups many of my clients have made.

I don't have time to eat lunch at work until 2 p.m., and by then I'm so hungry that I overeat!

Small Change Solution: If you've gone for more than four hours without fuel, of course you're going to want to overeat. It is crucial that you have a midmorning snack to tide you over. Keep a healthy morning "extra" on hand by making your morning snack a portable part of your breakfast prep. Bananas and a nonfat Greek-style yogurt (Greek-style yogurt is higher in protein than regular yogurt) are great options.

I am usually starved at 4 p.m., but I wait until I get home to eat.

Small Change Solution: If you have a busy job, especially one that involves intense face time with your computer, it can be hard to leave your desk during the workday. Unfortunately, skipping an afternoon snack when you are already starved will only ensure that you will overeat when you get home. Create a snack drawer in your desk, and keep it stocked for the week with snacks that don't need to be refrigerated. A piece of fruit (which can also satisfy a late-day sweet craving) with a serving of nuts, a whole-wheat crispbread spread with peanut butter, or a small bag of soy crisps could be a good choice.

After dinner, I can't stop eating.

Small Change Solution: Usually, if you skip meals or snacks during the day or you have gone long periods of time without eating, your body will try to catch up at night on what you missed. Look at the times you ate your meals and if there were any snacks. If this is your issue, make sure you're eating two balanced meals with two smart snacks before dinner, and your evening hunger will vanish with the last meal of the day.

In order for a snack to do its job, it must also be balanced. Otherwise you may still be hungry and just have wasted calories on food that didn't satisfy you. Think of a healthy snack as a *mini* meal (one that includes protein and carbs); portions should be smaller than at breakfast, lunch, or dinner. And chances are that this *mini* meal is not going to be found in the vending machine.

Small Change Snack Tips

1. Limit a snack to approximately 200 calories maximum.

2. Turn coffee or tea into a snack by adding a cup of low-fat milk or soymilk.

3. Do not have a carbohydrate alone (such as an apple or a serving of crackers); you will still be hungry. Instead, pair a carb with a lean protein or healthy fat. Have low-fat cheese with your apple, or some peanut butter on your whole grain crackers.

4. It's okay to have carbs alone before bed (such as a piece of fruit) because it doesn't need to keep you full—you're about to go to sleep.

5. Don't double dip. For instance, don't do string cheese and nuts, or string cheese and yogurt. Instead, choose one high-fiber carb and one lean protein or healthy fat; otherwise your calories (and fat) can add up.

6. When you eat straight from the bag, box, or can, you'll consume more. Preproportion items like nuts in resealable snack-size bags.

7. Try to keep snacktime to three hours after you have eaten. If you eat it too close to your last meal, it won't do its job for the next meal.

8. If buying an energy bar, read the label and look for more fiber and protein, less calories and fat.

9. Just because it's a "100-calorie pack" doesn't mean it is a healthy snack. Make sure it offers some fiber and protein or healthy fat—and if not, skip it.

Let's stop now and take a look at your food journal for the last two weeks. Have you changed your eating schedule? You don't need to be 100 percent perfect with this, or any small change, but you need to feel that this routine is becoming a part of who you are. At this point in your Small Change Plan, *the most important thing is that you are not skipping meals*. In other chapters, we will continue to work on improving the actual content of your meals. What counts now is that you're eating regularly.

YOU NEED THOSE ZZZZZS: THE LINK BETWEEN SLEEPING AND EATING

In order for your new routine of eating and not skipping meals to be truly successful, you need to get adequate sleep. What does sleeping have to do with healthy eating? If you don't get enough sleep, you are less likely to keep up with your new routine. Being overly tired can lead you to make poor decisions when you get up in the morning and you might fall back into old habits—the same habits, if you recall, that were not working for you.

If you are an evening owl, you end up eating more calories. You don't have to go to bed at 10 p.m. and get eight to nine hours of sleep per night; that might not be realistic for you. But take a close look at your sleep patterns. Most adults should aim for a minimum of seven hours. Personally, I do best with eight. A slight change with the amount of sleep you get, even finding just thirty minutes more per night, will help your body and your brain.

ARE YOU READY TO MOVE ON?

The Small Change Diet is about your personal success and your personal pace—no one else's. As you enjoy your new healthy-eating routine, you may enjoy immediate weight loss, but you will also be one step closer to a lifetime of health and weight loss. Take the Small Change Success Test below to see if you are ready to move on to the next change.

Small Change Success Test

1. Have you stopped skipping meals?

2. Are you eating at least one snack per day, at least between lunch and dinner?

3. Are you eating every three to four hours? And definitely not going more than five?

4. Are you getting at least seven hours of sleep?

If you answered yes to at least three of the items on this chapter's Small Change Success Test, you can handle another Small Change. If you find that you start to skip meals again, don't get frustrated—just get refocused.

Congratulations. It's time to move forward and tackle another Small Change!

SMALL CHANGE 2

▼▲▼▲▼▲▼▲▼

Brighten Your Plate, Naturally

More often than not, patients who come to me to lose weight don't eat enough fruits and veggies. They might have an apple with their lunch sandwich or a serving of broccoli at dinner, and that's about it for the day. Usually they tell me it is hard for them to find and keep fresh produce or it is too expensive. Sometimes, they just like their meats and carbs and they forget. Several of my patients even think they're going to lose weight by cutting the calories in fruit. Can you relate? Experts recommend that we eat two to four servings of fruit and three to five servings of veggies a day. But what most people don't know is that you're not only losing out on nutrients in a diet deficient in fruits and veggies, you are also missing out on one of the simplest weight-loss tricks.

To lose weight, look at fruits and veggies as healthy substitutions for what's currently on your plate. They are naturally low in calories and fat. Plus, the water and fiber they contain help fill you up, so you won't feel as hungry. Make five swaps a day—a cookie for an apple, less steak for a salad—you can easily cut 500 calories a day. Plus, you don't just lose weight, you also reduce your risk of diabetes, heart disease, and cancer. In addition to welcome fiber, vitamins, and minerals, fruits and veggies contain phytonutrients, plant-based compounds that research suggests help protect against many chronic diseases.

Most of my patients actually *like* fruits and veggies—they just don't know how to eat them regularly. Two to four servings of fruit really aren't a lot—eat one large banana, for example, and you can meet your minimum daily fruit quota. And three to five servings of veggies would surprise you—most large salads are enough. In this change, you'll learn plenty of ways to regularly add fruits and vegetables to your diet. But first we need to change the way you view your plate—literally.

THE PLATE MAKEOVER: BUILD YOUR MEALS WITH FRUITS AND VEGGIES

Meat and potatoes (or starchy foods like rice and pasta): For the average American, it's what's for dinner. The foods *themselves* aren't "bad"—plenty of thin people eat them, and so can you. The issue is balance. A plate built around meat and starch is out of balance, and plate after unbalanced plate leads to extra pounds around your waist and hips.

The solution is simple: Rebalance your plate. Build your meals around fruit and veggies rather than protein, fat, and carbs, and you will lose weight. To get back to balance, use the Healthy Plate method:

1. Fill half your plate with nonstarchy veggies, such as broccoli, kale, steamed zucchini, or green beans. Starchy veggies like peas and corn contain more calories and thus should take up a little less than half your plate. (Refer to page 52 for exact serving sizes.)

2. Fill one-quarter of your plate with high-fiber and whole-grain choices: brown rice, whole-wheat pasta, quinoa, whole-wheat couscous, barley, oats, a serving of whole-wheat bread, or a baked potato/sweet potato.

3. Fill one-quarter of your plate with lean protein: skinless poultry, beans, fish, tofu, egg whites, low-fat dairy, pork tenderloins, or lean beef (i.e., sirloin).

4. If you are still hungry, enjoy a piece of fruit for dessert.

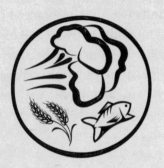

Don't be surprised if you rediscover how tasty and convenient fruits and veggies can be and you go over your minimum servings. As long as you use them to replace high-calorie, high-fat foods, you're doing great.

Your Small Change Plan

1. Eat a serving of fruit at breakfast.

2. Add veggies and/or fruit to lunch.

3. Start dinner with a salad.

4. Add a veggie to dinner.

5. Snack on one piece of fruit a day.

HAVE A BERRY GOOD MORNING!

When Matt, thirty-eight, first came to my office, he was finding it very hard to lose weight. He claimed he succeeded many times before, but this time, for some reason, he was lacking the discipline he needed to make it happen. I did a 24-recall with him and discovered that he was drinking a lot of fruit juice and not eating any whole fruits, among other diet disasters.

Matt began to include a piece of fruit with his breakfast. Eventually, he added another piece as a snack and decreased his juice intake. A year after his first visit and changing his behaviors, he is fifty pounds lighter.

As Matt discovered, adding fruit to breakfast is a sweet way to start your day, and it's so simple—just add berries to your cereal, top your toast with a tablespoon of almond or peanut butter and sliced banana, or whip up a smoothie with your favorite fruit. (Of course, be mindful of serving sizes—use the list on pages 50–51.)

I love fresh fruit myself—I enjoy fresh raspberries so much I buy them year round. If you opt for fresh fruit, make sure there are no bruises or spots. It should smell fresh, and be either ripe enough to eat right away or in a few days. And no matter which type of fruit you buy, wash it before you eat it. There's no need to buy special fruit and vegetable washes. Simply rub fruit briskly under running water to remove dirt and surface microorganisms, and then dry it.

Frozen or canned fruit can be just as nutritious, provided you make the right choices.

Fresh, Frozen, or Canned? Whatever You'll Eat!

My philosophy is simple: fruits and veggies first and foremost. I don't care whether you eat fresh, frozen, or canned fruits and veggies, as long as you eat them. Which one you choose depends on your lifestyle and budget.

If you prefer the taste of fresh produce, that's great. Just know that once it's picked, heat, light, and time break down some of its nutrients. So the amount of nutrients in that fresh spinach in your crisper, or those pears on your counter, depends on how long ago they were picked, how many days they spent in transit to your supermarket, and how long they sat before you ate them. For the greatest nutritional value and flavor, buy produce in season, from your local farmers' market or roadside stand.

If cost and convenience are your top concerns,

it's fine to opt for frozen or canned fruit and veggies, which are generally processed immediately upon harvest when their nutrient content is at its peak. The variety is very good, especially in frozen fruits. For example, it's a good bet that you'll find mango and papaya chunks in your frozen-foods aisle.

To trim calories, opt for fruits packed in their own juice, rather than heavy syrups. If you watch your sodium intake, choose veggies canned without added salt. If you already have canned veggies with added salt in your pantry, simply drain the packing liquid through a colander and rinse the vegetable under cold water for around two minutes.

As a dietitian, I've heard every fruit cop-out:

I don't like fruit.

Small Change Solution: Not even blueberries? Or bananas? Most people like more than one type of fruit, but if you really truly like only one, then eat only that one. Eating a variety of fruits and veggies is certainly a commendable goal, but as a realist, I'd rather have you eat just one type of fruit than skip it altogether.

I only like berries, but they're not in season year round.

Small Change Solution: Sure they are, if you buy them frozen. Thaw or microwave one serving and add them to your cereal or to a breakfast smoothie. They won't have the texture of fresh, in-season berries, but they will definitely have the flavor.

It's so expensive!

Small Change Solution: Not if you buy in season and local. Come spring, you can feast on rhubarb and strawberries. In the summer, you'll find just-picked berries of all types, melons fresh from local fields, as well as peaches and nectarines. In the fall, you can crunch into apples from local orchards; plus figs, grapes, and ruby red pomegranates are in season. Visit your local farmers' market to get good buys. Winter means citrus—oranges, grapefruit, and tangerines. If your favorite fruit (including tropical fruit, such as mangos) doesn't grow in your region, or is out of season, chances are you can still find it in the produce aisle or in the frozen-foods section.

Small Change Fruit Breakfast Tips

1. Buy plain, low-fat cottage cheese and add your fruit of choice.

2. When berries are out of season, buy them frozen. To thaw them fast, put one serving in the microwave for two or three minutes, then stir them into plain low-fat yogurt.

3. To add natural sweetness to your morning oatmeal, slice a pear, apple, or banana into it and then cook it.

4. Top high-fiber breakfast cereal with a cup of berries instead of added sugar.

5. For a quick, hearty on-the-run breakfast, make a peanut butter and banana sandwich.

ADD SOME PRODUCE TO YOUR MIDDAY MEAL

Think about it. What's a typical American lunch? A sandwich with chips, a burger with fries, maybe a slice or two of pizza? The average person is not used to eating fruit or veggies for lunch. Many of my patients weren't either. However, they have found it to be easier and more convenient than they'd thought. Some solutions are absurdly simple. For example, you can top your sandwich with lettuce (or darker, nutritious spinach leaves), tomatoes, and other veggies, and end your lunch with a serving of fruit—berries, watermelon, kiwi, an apple or banana, whatever you like.

What's true for fruit is also true of veggies: fresh is always great, if you can get it or you don't mind the prep work. Select green leafy veggies that are springy (not wilted), and in general choose veggies with bright color and crispness. As I said, frozen or canned veggies can be just as nutritious, as long as you don't smother them in butter, gravy, cheese, or sauces. Buy organic produce if you like, and wash all veggies thoroughly.

While adding fruits and veggies to lunch is easier than you think, let's dispense with any lingering doubts.

My cafeteria doesn't serve veggies.

Small Change Solution: Since you'll soon be eating veggies with dinner, too, prepare an extra serving, and bring it with you to add to your lunch. To make it easy to bring veggies from home, buy those single-serving plastic containers with lids—they're typically right next to the plastic bags and aluminum foil in the supermarket. You might also make a side salad at a local deli or supermarket that has a salad bar to have with your sandwich.

My sandwich is very filling and I don't have room for fruit or veggies.

Small Change Solution: My guess is that you're full because your sandwich contains too much meat, cheese, or other added fats (mayo in chicken salad, etc.). By contrast, a serving of fruit or a side salad is lower in calories, and their fiber can help fill you up, too. Simply reduce the high-calorie fillings so you have room to build your meal with fruit and vegetables.

I love French fries—aren't they a vegetable?

Small Change Solution: I love them, too. Sadly, although a potato is theoretically a vegetable, when I refer to "veggies," I don't include potatoes. That's because they're much higher in calories than all of the others. So I count them as a starch only. That doesn't mean you can't eat French fries, though. It simply means that you can't count them as a veggie.

Small Change Veggie/Fruit Lunch Tips

1. Build your sandwich with lettuce, tomato, cucumber, and onions instead of more meat or cheese.

2. Order a side salad with diet or low-fat dressing with a sandwich or burger instead of French fries.

3. Bring some baby carrots and celery sticks to munch on with your lunch.

4. If you are having a salad as your entrée for lunch, consider adding some orange, pear, or apple slices to help fill you up.

5. Bring a piece of fruit for dessert.

A SINGLE SERVING

Whether you're talking about fruits or veggies, relax—serving sizes are small. Remember, your goal is to consume two to four servings of fruit and three to five servings of veggies per day. Below is what is considered a "single serving."

Fruit

- Apple: 1 small (4 ounces)
- Applesauce (unsweetened): ½ cup
- Banana: 1 medium (4 inches)
- Blueberries: ¾ cup

- Cantaloupe or honeydew: 1 cup cubed
- Cherries: 12
- Fruit cocktail (own juice only): ½ cup
- Grapefruit: ½ medium
- Grapes: 17 small
- Juices (100 percent fruit): 4 to 6 ounces
- Kiwifruit: 1 (3½ ounces)
- Orange: 1 medium
- Peach: 1 medium
- Plums: 2 small
- Prunes: 3
- Raisins and other dried fruit: 2 tablespoons
- Raspberries: 1 cup
- Strawberries (whole): 1¼ cups
- Watermelon: 1 cup balls

Veggies

Although you'll find serving sizes for the veggies listed on the next page, feel free to eat as many as you wish, as long as they're not prepared with fat (i.e., butter, cheese, oil). With starchy veggies like peas and corn, stick to the recommended serving sizes.

- Cooked or chopped raw veggies (asparagus, brussels sprouts, broccoli, carrots, cauliflower, celery, cucumber, green beans, leeks, onions, peppers, zucchini): ½ cup

- Corn: ½ cup cooked or 1 medium ear

- Mixed veggies: ½ cup

- Peas: ½ cup

- Raw leafy veggies (kale, romaine and all lettuce, spinach, watercress): 1 cup

- Squash (acorn, butternut, winter): 1 cup

✔ How's It Going?

Are you learning about your eating patterns from your food journal? Are you able to translate what you've learned into positive action?

START DINNER WITH A SALAD

Whether you're eating in or dining out, this small change is crucial. It's an opportunity to fill yourself up as well as add fiber and other nutrients to your meal. If you already include a side salad with dinner, wonderful! If you don't, it's time to start, because as long as you don't use high-calorie toppings and dressings, salads are low on calories and high on satisfying fiber. They're also delicious.

But let's not forget: A salad is built with veggies. Begin with a cup of leafy greens, which are rich in folate, a B vitamin needed for the growth of healthy cells. The darker the greens, the better (but if you don't like them, don't use them). Then add bright-hued veggies—tomatoes, carrots, cucumbers, and red, yellow, or orange bell peppers. The more color-ful the veggies, the more health-promoting phyto-chemicals they contain.

I've worked with patients who love salad (but just forget to eat it) and those who dislike it (but then get used to it). Among the most common salad sob stories I hear:

I hate dark leafy greens!

Small Change Solution: Then don't eat them. The point of eating a side salad before dinner is to help fill you up, so you eat less protein, starchy carbohydrates, and fat. If you only like iceberg let-tuce, that's fine by me. (Every once in a while, I enjoy a wedge salad—which is always made with iceberg lettuce—dressed with balsamic vinaigrette instead of the standard blue cheese.) Or, if you just hate salads in general, double up on your veggies at dinner.

I don't have time to make a salad.

Small Change Solution: I hear this a lot. My response is always, "How long does it take to pop open a bag of lettuce, throw it in a bowl, and add a few grape tomatoes?" Washed, bagged lettuce, and prewashed, precut salad veggies are there for time-pressed folks like you. Use them.

Low-calorie diet dressings taste terrible!

Small Change Solution: If you think they taste terrible, don't use them. Or maybe you just haven't found the right low-calorie dressing. In any event, make sure you use the correct serving size (generally 2 tablespoons) and pass up any other added fats in your salad (i.e., cheese, bacon bits, and croutons). Another trick: Put the dressing on the side, dip your fork in the dressing, then spear up your lettuce and veggies; if you used to ladle on the blue-cheese or Thousand Island dressing, you'll save hundreds of calories without denying yourself the taste you love.

Small Change Salad Tips

1. Slice and chop enough veggies (i.e., cucumber, onion) for two or three days of salads.

2. If you find the taste of greens bland, sprinkle them with a tablespoon of tangy feta or Parmesan cheese (adds a lot of flavor for not a lot of calories or fat).

3. If you miss the crunch of croutons, top your salad with a tablespoon of chopped almonds, walnuts, or sunflower seeds.

4. When you can't muster the will even to tear open a bag of prewashed greens, make your side salad at your supermarket's salad bar. You'll pay for the convenience, but you'll also stick to your healthy eating plan, and that's priceless.

5. If you're starving when you get home from work, prepare your salad, eat it, and then cook the rest of your meal.

SHOULD YOU GO ORGANIC?

Must you? Absolutely not—nonorganic fruits and veggies are just as nutritious. But if you're concerned about the pesticides used on produce, consider this: If you avoid the top twelve most pesticide-laden fruits and veggies (the "Dirty Dozen"), you can lower your exposure to pesticides by almost 90 percent, according to the Environmental Working Group (EWG), a nonprofit research organization based in Washington, D.C., that has been publishing guides to the "Dirty Dozen" of most contaminated foods since 1995, based on statistical analyses of testing by the USDA and the FDA.

That's what I do—if I want, say, apples or bell peppers, I buy the organic variety if it's available or select another fruit or veggie that's lower on the list. (Washing and peeling may reduce levels of some pesticides, but not all.) Still, if I want spinach for dinner and organic is not available, I'll go with the nonorganic variety. It's more important to get in those fruits and veggies.

Highest in Pesticides
Consider organic when buying

1. Celery

2. Peaches

3. Strawberries

4. Apples

5. Blueberries (domestic)

6. Nectarines

7. Sweet bell peppers

8. Spinach

9. Cherries

10. Kale / Collard greens

11. Potatoes

12. Grapes (imported)

Lowest in Pesticides (the "Clean 15")
Nonorganic is fine when buying

1. Onions

2. Avocado

3. Sweet corn (frozen)

4. Pineapple

5. Mango

6. Sweet peas (frozen)

7. Asparagus

8. Kiwi

9. Cabbage

10. Eggplant

11. Cantaloupe

12. Watermelon

13. Grapefruit

14. Sweet potatoes

15. Honeydew melon

INVITE A VEGGIE TO DINNER

One of my patients, Julie, forty-five, complained to me that she couldn't lose weight like she used to. We reviewed her weekly food journal to find that she wasn't eating enough veggies, especially at dinner. Typically, her plate held either chicken or meat, along with either rice or potato, but no veggie.

"I really don't love that many veggies," she said. We chatted about what veggies she *did* like, and she said that carrots and peas were her favorite. I encouraged her to include them with dinner and reduce the other servings on her plate.

Two weeks later, she had dropped four pounds. By adding more veggies to her dinner plate, she was able to reduce the amount of protein and starch she was consuming to feel full and started saving calories without realizing it.

So don't focus on the veggies you don't like.

Just eat the ones you do like. For example, if you plan on pasta, top it with ratatouille, a kind of veggie stew that originated in the Provençal region of France. Tomatoes are a key ingredient, along with zucchini, eggplant, bell peppers, carrots, and spices. The more room for veggies, the less room for the pasta.

Also, think of the produce section as an uncharted island—it can seem that way for those who don't like vegetables—and yourself as an adventurer. Explore the produce section, frozen-foods section, or canned veggie aisle for vegetables you'd like to try, whether fancy heirloom tomatoes, canned artichokes, collard greens, frozen baby brussels sprouts, or sugar snap peas.

I'd also encourage you to scour the Internet for interesting low-fat, low-calorie veggie recipes that you can make in fifteen minutes or less. If you can put a pot of water on the stove, and put a steamer on top of that, voilà—steamed veggies. If you can place cut-up mushrooms, zucchini, onions, and red peppers on a baking tray, and then spray them with canola oil spray, you can make roasted vegetables. Add some herbs and spices—rosemary, salt, pepper, garlic, balsamic vinegar—and you're well on your way to knowing how to prepare them in tasty and waist-trimming ways.

Of course, there are many excuses associated with veggies. Moms the world over have heard them all, and so have I.

I hate veggies!

Small Change Solution: I hear this a lot, but sorry, you're an adult now, and when was the last time you actually tried eating veggies? You have more choices than the boiled, overcooked broccoli you might be familiar with. Try roasting veggies—carrots, brightly colored red peppers, and zucchini take on a richer, sweeter flavor—or top them with a bit of grated Parmesan. Mash steamed cauliflower with a teaspoon of olive oil, or lightly sauté spinach with a bit of minced garlic.

I only like "bad" vegetables, like peas and corn.

Small Change Solution: I really wish people would stop thinking of food as "bad." There are only better choices! If you really, really want a serving of corn or peas, go for it, because there is not a vegetable in the world that is "bad" for you. Just watch your serving sizes, and don't drown them in a sea of butter, cheese, or other fatty extras.

Veggies are a waste of money; I buy them then watch them go bad.

Small Change Solution: Have you seen the pre-washed, already cut-up veggies in the supermarket produce aisle? They're there because the supermarket execs know that many people don't have the time, energy, or patience to wash, peel, and slice veggies. And you'll actually eat the prepped veggies, so they're worth the extra buck. Or take the cheaper option: Buy frozen or canned veggies, which are just as nutritious and fresh.

Small Change Veggie-with-Dinner Tips

1. Buy frozen veggies in a microwavable bag for convenience.

2. Cook extra veggies tonight to have leftovers for tomorrow night, and you've cut your veggie prep time in half.

3. Throw chopped veggies (i.e., broccoli, eggplant, and zucchini) into tomato sauce for pasta.

4. If you don't enjoy steamed veggies, try roasting them with a touch of olive oil.

5. To flavor veggies without extra fat and calories, give them a squeeze of lemon or a drizzle of balsamic vinegar, or top them with a tablespoon of salsa or a heaping teaspoon of Parmesan.

SNACK ON ONE PIECE OF FRUIT A DAY

As revealed in Small Change 1, I tell my patients to eat two snacks a day—one between breakfast and lunch, and another between lunch and dinner. When it comes to weight loss, snacks are crucial: Not only do they help fuel your body between meals, they head off poor choices at your next meal. I also view snacks as an opportunity to have fruit, which most people don't get enough of in their diets. Fruit is a great part of a healthy snack because it's nutritious *and* filling.

It's also delicious. Sweet, creamy bananas . . . tart, crunchy apples . . . juicy blueberries or black-berries. There's a fruit out there that you love—or at least like—and whatever it is, it makes the perfect snack. Fruit is versatile, too. You can eat it whole when you're on the go, or slice it and dress it with a low-cal dressing (yogurt and cin-namon . . . yum). You can even grill it! In the fall and winter, enjoy a baked apple or poached pear, or fry a banana in butter-flavored cooking spray, which will satisfy your sweet tooth and craving for comfort food.

There are a variety of reasons my patients give for not snacking on fruit. Among the most common:

I always forget.

Small Change Solution: One of fruit's many virtues is that so many varieties are portable—perfect for occjur car-centric, hectic lives. While pomegranates and pineapple don't fit the bill, apples, oranges, pears, and bananas are pretty easy to eat on your way out the door, or keep on your desk at the office.

Fruit is too much work—I hate all the peeling and cutting.

Small Change Solution: Most supermarkets—and now many convenience stores—offer fruit cups filled with fresh berries, grapes, watermelon, pineapple, melon, and even kiwi. You'll pay a bit more, but you will more than likely meet your daily fruit quota. Or you could buy frozen or canned fruit. Thaw one serving of melon or berries, or open a can of fruit packed in its own juice, and you're done.

Snacking on fruit makes me hungry.

Small Change Solution: You're right, it does. That's because fruit is primarily carbohydrate, and eating carbs alone won't satisfy your hunger; you digest carbs the quickest, protein and fat slower. To give fruit that stick-to-your-ribs quality, pair it with a small amount of protein, which digests slower than carbs and has a high satiety factor—in other words, it satisfies hunger. Good protein options: an ounce of cheese, ½ cup of cottage cheese, or an ounce of nuts.

Small Change Fruit-as-a-Snack Tips

1. Buy an extra piece of fruit with your breakfast and save it for your snack.

2. As with breakfast, add whole fruit to protein-rich plain yogurt for a delicious and filling snack.

3. If you're pressed for time, buy your fruit already cut up (i.e., pineapple, melon, or strawberries) and enjoy with a serving of nuts.

4. Every morning, pack a piece of string cheese and a serving of fruit (either whole or sliced) to snack on in the afternoon.

5. After dinner, snack on one serving of fruit. (Don't worry about adding protein here, since you ideally don't need it to hold you over since it should be close to bedtime.)

ARE YOU READY TO MOVE ON?

Remember, I want you to progress at your own pace. If you were a fruit and veggie lover before, this Small Change—snacking on fruit or adding a salad to dinner—might have been relatively simple. But if your diet was seriously lacking in produce, it may take more time to acquire the habit, and it will probably produce more results. Either way, it's okay—you're on your way, and that's what counts. Take the following Small Change Success Test to see if you are ready to move on to the next Small Change.

Small Change Success Test

1. Are you eating a serving of fruit at breakfast?

2. Are you adding veggies and/or fruit to your lunch?

3. Are you starting your dinner with a salad?

4. Have you added a vegetable to your dinner?

5. Do you snack on one piece of fruit a day?

If you answered yes to at least three of these questions, add one more Small Change. If you're still working on making more than two of these Small Changes, be patient and keep trying. You'll get there!

If you've answered yes to four or five questions, congratulations. It's time to tackle another Small Change!

Think Before You Drink (Sip, Guzzle, or Chug)

When Frank, twenty-seven, first came to see me, he weighed 240 pounds—40 more than he needed—and drank lots of soda, every day. He told me that he also ate a lot of fast food, sometimes more than once per day, and had acquired the habit of ordering a 32-ounce soda with his meals. He struggled for weeks to rein in his cola habit, couldn't do it, and didn't lose weight. Six weeks later, however, he'd managed to halve his cola intake, swapped it for water, and lost two pounds. A month after that, he'd quit completely, and lost another six pounds. Eight pounds gone in ten weeks—just from giving up soda!

Frank's story shows how fattening soda and other sweetened beverages can be. Americans consume just over 22 teaspoons of added sugars per day, government nutrition surveys show. At 16 calories per teaspoon, 22 teaspoons of sugar contain about 355 calories—and most of this sugar is consumed in beverages, including soda, juices, and energy and coffee drinks. These sugary beverages contain mostly empty calories that don't satisfy the appetite. As a result, people consume more fluid calories in an attempt to get full. In fact, some studies suggest that when you *drink* too many calories, you're more likely to gain weight than if you *eat* too many.

Many people don't realize just how many calories their favorite beverages might add to their total daily intake. While the calories in all beverages are listed right on the Nutrition Facts label, you need to make a distinction between a serving and the contents of the entire cup, can, or bottle. For example, the label on the 20-ounce bottle of your favorite drink might say that an 8-ounce serving contains 100 calories. However, the *bottle* contains 20 ounces—that's 2.5 servings. So while one "serving" of your drink is indeed 100 calories, you'll consume 250 calories if you drink the whole bottle—and most people do!

What's more, the sweeteners that add calories to beverages go by so many different names, you might not recognize them. Besides plain "sugar," common sweeteners include high-fructose corn syrup, fructose, fruit juice concentrates, honey, sucrose, and dextrose. If these ingredients are on the label, the beverage contains sugar.

Water is the ultimate health drink, and we all need to drink enough of it (more on that in a moment). However, variety is a wonderful thing, and if you drink your favorite beverages in moderation, they won't affect your health or waistline.

How to reduce the number of calories you drink? "Beverage awareness" is the first step. Read the Nutrition Facts label on cans and bottles carefully, read the nutrition information listed on company websites, and record your daily beverages in your food journal, so you can see for yourself how many calories they add to your daily intake. Before long, you'll learn to make small but smart choices that allow you to drink your favorite beverages, rather than wear them around your hips.

FIRST THINGS FIRST: GET THE FLUID YOU NEED

Every day you lose water, both in the bathroom and through your breath and perspiration. For your body to function properly, you must consume drinks and foods that contain water.

Water itself is your best bet because it's inexpensive, everywhere, and calorie free. You have other healthy options, though. Milk and 100 percent fruit juice are mostly water. So are beer, wine, and caffeinated beverages (coffee, tea, soda), although they shouldn't count as a major portion of your daily fluid total. Foods contain water, too, especially fruits and veggies like watermelon and tomatoes. In fact, water from food provides about 20 percent of the average person's total daily fluid intake.

Beyond health, fluids play a key role in weight control. If you don't drink enough fluid, you may feel tired, mentally foggy . . . and hungry. Yes, dehydration is often mistaken for hunger. To find out if you're hungry or simply thirsty, drink a glass of water and wait a few minutes. If your hunger fades, you were thirsty, even if you didn't feel thirsty.

The amount of fluid you need each day varies. Although the "eight eight-ounce glasses a day" recommendation is a good guide, you may need more or less, depending on your size, health, activity level, and climate.

I use a general formula: 1 ounce of fluid for every 30 calories you consume. That means if you're a smaller and/or sedentary woman who consumes about 1,400 calories a day, you'd need to consume about six cups of fluid. If you consume 2,000 calories a day, considered the "average" intake, you'd need that standard eight cups. If you're a large man, or very physically active, and consume 2,500 calories, you need ten cups a day. You'd also need more in special circumstances, which include pregnancy and breastfeeding, illnesses that cause vomiting and diarrhea, heavy exercise, summer heat, or a hot, dry climate.

Your Small Change Plan

1. Aim for eight cups of fluids, with an emphasis on water, a day.

2. Sip seltzer water or club soda instead of regular soda.

3. Switch from whole milk to 1 percent low-fat or nonfat milk.

4. If you drink juice or fruit drinks, opt for 100 percent fruit juice, and limit it to eight ounces a day.

5. Switch from "fancy" sugar-sweetened coffee or tea drinks to regular coffee or tea. It is always better to add your own sugar, if needed, to control amount.

6. If you drink alcohol, stick to one to two glasses of wine or beer, or one cocktail a day.

WATER: THE ULTIMATE "ENERGY DRINK"

You want to lose weight, right? Then water is your friend. It really does fill you up, and may help prevent you from filling out. In a study conducted at Virginia Polytechnic Institute and State University, researchers found that postmenopausal women who drank 1.5 cups of water before a meal reported that they felt fuller. As a result, they consumed about 60 fewer calories than those who didn't drink water before a meal. If you think 60 calories isn't much, try this strategy every day for a year. You'll save a total of 21,900 calories, which is the equivalent of six pounds!

Okay, not everyone likes the taste of plain water. Many, it seems, are my patients, who inevitably ask if it's okay to drink those vitamin or flavored waters. Sure, if they're less than 25 calories per cup (some brands contain no calories at all). If they contain more calories than that, watch out! Some flavored waters are packed with sugar, and hence calories. Read the Nutrition Facts label. If the bottle contains more beverage than the serving size, shop around for a lower-calorie brand.

I've heard every excuse in the book for why people don't reach for water more often. Here are the most common.

I honestly don't like the taste of water.

Small Change Solution: Who says you have to drink it plain? Dress it up. Flavor your water with a wedge of lemon or lime, fresh mint, or a few slices of cucumber. Or try fruit-flavored seltzer water, which packs a lot of flavor into zero calories and appeals even to those who simply can't take plain water.

I forget to drink it.

Small Change Solution: So do I, especially when I don't keep a water bottle on my desk. Try it—you can't forget when a bottle or glass is right there in front of you. You might also put sticky notes that say "drink up" where you're sure to see them—on your desktop or laptop or on the refrigerator door. Soon enough, you'll remember to drink your water regularly.

I just don't get thirsty.

Small Change Solution: That doesn't mean your body doesn't need water and other fluids. Dehydration occurs when your body doesn't have enough water to carry out normal functions. Even mild dehydration can drain your energy and fog your thinking. If you're urinating less than usual, or if you rarely feel thirsty, check the color of your urine.

If it's straw colored, you're properly hydrated. If it's dark, you're dehydrated—drink up, whether you're thirsty or not.

Small Change Water Tips

1. Drink a glass of water before each meal.

2. When you dine out, "order" a glass of water as soon as you're seated.

3. Keep a bottle of water on your desk at work as a reminder to drink up.

4. If you're conscious of the environment and/or the cost of bottled water, get your own container and fill it from home.

5. Keep water in your purse, briefcase, or backpack so you can hydrate on the run.

SODA: LIQUID CALORIES YOU DON'T NEED

I have a hard time telling my patients that it's okay to drink soda. Yes, it counts toward your daily fluid intake, but it's a waste of calories. Consider the ingredients in a 20-ounce bottle of cola. You get carbonated water, artificial flavor, caffeine, and about 17 teaspoons of sugar (250 calories). Even a smaller 12-ounce can contains about 150 calories, 10 teaspoons of sugar, and no nutrients at all. Let's not even get into the calories contained in one 32- or 44-ounce supersized soda.

Here's another way to look at how soda affects your weight. (I've done the math so you don't have to.) If you drink one can a day for a year, you consume about 55,000 calories in soda alone. (It takes 3,500 calories to equal one pound of body weight.) That means that one 12-ounce soda a day translates into 16 pounds of extra weight over one year! If you drink one 20-ounce bottle of soda (which contains about 250 calories), you'll drink up about 91,000 calories, which translates into 26 pounds of extra weight!

If you drink sweetened soda, be brave and give it up—you will find it much easier to cut calories and lose weight. You need to consume 500 calories less per day to lose one pound a week (again, 3,500 calories = one pound). If you drink two 20-ounce bottles of soda a day, and cut them out of your diet, you'll save 500 calories right there. Boom—one pound gone.

Diet soda is the obvious alternative to the sugar-sweetened kind. The general consensus in the scientific community is that artificial sweeteners are safe, so one or two diet sodas a day is fine. If they're your sole source of fluids throughout the day, however, mix it up a bit. Water is a great option. So are seltzer water and club soda. (The only difference between these clear, bubbly beverages is that club soda contains 50 milligrams of sodium per serving, while seltzer does not.) Avoid tonic water, which contains 83 calories and 22 grams of sugar, as well as 25 grams of sodium.

Here's more food for thought. Those sodas, juices, fancy coffee drinks, and other sugar-sweetened beverages don't just make your jeans snug. Evidence suggests that drinking too many of them may also threaten your health.

In one Harvard study that followed 88,000 women for twenty-four years, those who drank at least two sugar-sweetened drinks a day had a 20 percent higher risk of heart disease, compared with those who drank less than one sugary drink a month, regardless of their body weight.

In another study among 4,000 men and women who participated in the prestigious Framingham Heart Study for four years, those who drank at least one sugar-sweetened soft drink a day faced a 44 percent greater risk of metabolic syndrome, a precursor of heart disease and diabetes, compared to those who drank less. Again, the risk was independent of their weight. So cut back on sugary drinks, and you'll likely trim your risk of chronic disease along with your waistline.

I know it's hard to give up soda, because I've heard the reasons for this time and again.

I've had soda with my meals since I was a kid.

Small Change Solution: It's time to outgrow that habit . . . either that or outgrow your clothes. Many people wean themselves off regular soda by switching to diet. While you may not like it at first, you'll get used to it. If it's strictly the bubbles you're after, switch to plain or flavored seltzer, club soda, or water—plain or flavored in the ways I suggested earlier.

I would switch to diet soda, but don't artificial sweeteners cause cancer?

Small Change Solution: The claims that artificial sweeteners can cause numerous health problems, including cancer, are persistent and scary. However, there simply isn't scientific evidence to support them. According to the National Cancer Institute, there's no evidence that any of the artificial sweeteners approved for use in the United States cause cancer, and numerous studies confirm that artificial sweeteners are safe for the general population. Virtually the only people who cannot consume the artificial sweetener aspartame are those who have a rare hereditary disease called phenylketonuria (PKU)—and every product that contains aspartame carries a PKU warning on the label.

I don't like the taste of club soda or seltzer.

Small Change Solution: If you're committed to losing weight, you'll give them another try—you never know what you can develop a taste for! Flavor them with wedges of lemon or lime, as I suggested earlier, or stick to plain water.

Small Change Soda Tips

1. If you currently drink soda, cut back gradually over a two-week period. For example, if you now drink five cans per day, go to four, then three, and so on until you're off it completely.

2. Experiment with alternatives to soda that aren't sweetened with sugar and contain 25 calories or less per serving—iced or hot herbal teas, for example.

3. Limit diet sodas to one or two a day. Then switch to seltzer or club soda.

4. Don't keep soda in the house.

5. Enjoy one serving of regular soda on a special occasion, like at a ball game (as long as you don't have season tickets).

MILK: SIP THE NUTRIENTS, SKIP THE FAT

Rich in calcium, vitamin D, protein, and other nutrients, milk gives you a lot of bang for your buck, nutritionally speaking. What no one needs, though, is the saturated fat and extra calories in whole milk. Diets high in saturated fats are linked to high blood cholesterol and heart disease, and one cup of whole milk contains three times as much saturated fat as the same amount of low-fat milk—4.6 grams of saturated fat in whole milk versus 1.5 grams in low-fat milk.

If you currently drink whole milk, think of your heart as well as your hips, and make the switch to low-fat milk. The best thing about low-fat milk: The fat is gone but the nutrients remain. To ease the transition, move from whole milk to 2 percent, then to 1 percent, and finally to nonfat over two weeks or a month. (During the transition period, buy quarts of milk, rather than gallons, so you won't waste it.) If you really hate the taste of nonfat milk, you can stop at 1 percent. Or try "skim plus" milk—skim milk with milk proteins added. The result is a much thicker, creamier "skim," without the extra fat and calories.

When it comes to milk, I've found that people either love it or hate it. But low-fat milk is so good for you, and with evidence that low-fat dairy may promote weight loss, you owe it to yourself to rise above the most common excuses for avoiding it.

I'm lactose intolerant.

Small Change Solution: Then you're likely familiar with lactose-free milk. If you haven't tried it, give it a chance. Not only does it taste sweeter than regular milk, it provides the same important nutrients as regular milk and comes in 1 percent and nonfat varieties.

Isn't milk fattening?

Small Change Solution: As I mentioned earlier, while whole milk contains a significant amount of fat, the nonfat variety does not—and is filled with nutrients to boot. Also, milk is an excellent source of protein, which when included as part of a meal or snack can help fill you up. As long as you stick with 8-ounce serving sizes, milk can fit into a healthy diet.

I only like chocolate or strawberry milk.

Small Change Solution: You don't have to give them up. Just opt for the low-fat variety. While flavored milks do contain added sugar, you still benefit from milk's nutrients. After lunch, for dessert, I mix four ounces of nonfat milk with four ounces of low-fat chocolate milk. I call it a "milk swirl"—yum!

Small Change Milk Tips

1. Switch from whole milk to lower fat varieties gradually over a period of a week or two.

2. If you don't enjoy the taste of plain milk, try flavored low-fat milk or mix plain milk with the flavored kind.

3. For a warm and healthy drink, steam a cup of low-fat or nonfat milk and add a dash of vanilla and cinnamon.

4. Eat cereal for breakfast, if you don't now, so you can consume about a cup of milk that way.

5. Slip milk into a smoothie—use ½ cup nonfat milk, ½ cup nonfat yogurt, and a cup of berries.

SPORTS DRINKS: WHEN YOU NEED
'EM, WHEN YOU DON'T

Sports drinks are great—for athletes. These beverages, which commonly contain sugar and other sweeteners, delay fatigue and increase endurance. But not everyone with a gym membership needs them, and those who drink them unnecessarily may derail their weight-loss efforts.

As a general rule, if you perform endurance exercise, or are in training for a sporting event like a marathon or triathlon, sports drinks can help—they'll supply your body with the fluids and electrolytes it needs and replenish its supply of glucose. If your workout is relatively easy, however—a 30- to 45-minute walk or jog or a normal strength-training session—you probably don't need them, especially if you're trying to lose weight. The 150 sweetened calories (or more) they contain will likely cancel out the calories you burn.

While you don't need a sports drink's extra calories to pedal an elliptical trainer or pump iron, you still need to stay hydrated, especially if you work out in a hot, humid room or climate. In this situation, water is the perfect "energy drink." Or try one of the newer sports drinks that are lower in sugar, and therefore lower in calories. Opt for those with around 25 calories per eight-ounce serving, or a brand with 0 calories. Read those Nutrition Facts labels, and you'll find one—even athletes want to cut back on sugar!

FRUIT JUICE: GO NATURAL!

There are lots of "fruit juices" on the market, and most contain a lot of added sweeteners. Those extra calories can cause weight gain, especially if you drink fruit juice throughout the day.

If you drink it, check the ingredients on the Nutrition Facts label. If it contains added sweeteners, opt for a variety that says it is (not contains) "100 percent fruit juice," with no added sugar (or high-fructose corn syrup, or honey, or any other sweetener). While 100 percent fruit juice may contain about the same number of calories as sweetened fruit drinks, you will get more vitamins and nutrients and fewer additives from 100 percent juice.

One serving size of 100 percent fruit juice, which is eight ounces, fits into a well-balanced diet. If you typically drink more juice than that, cut those eight ounces with seltzer, water, or club soda. It's a refreshing, tasty way to make your daily fluid quota, and you can use any fruit juice you like, as long as it's 100 percent juice. I use this trick myself—I love orange juice, so I mix one part OJ to three parts seltzer.

Although you might love juice, don't totally

exclude fruit for juice, especially when you have a snack. For example, a whole apple contains more fiber than eight ounces of 100 percent apple juice, and fiber can help fill you up.

Here are some common fruit juice misunderstandings:

I thought juice was good for me.

Small Change Solution: Well, 100 percent fruit juice is, but it's still high in calories. Whether you eat excess calories or drink them, the end result is weight gain.

It's easier to drink fruit juice than to eat fruit.

Small Change Solution: Is it easier to go out and buy new clothes, in bigger sizes, than to wear the ones you have? Get in the habit of eating your calories rather than drinking them. Bananas, apples, pears, and berries are all easy to eat. So are the fruit cups you can buy at the supermarket.

Small Change Fruit Juice Tips

1. Select only 100 percent fruit juice. Read every brand's Nutrition Facts label, and pass up those that contain added sugar or other sweeteners.

2. "Cut" your juice with seltzer, club soda, or water.

3. Once you've reached your daily eight-ounce juice quota, reach for a piece of whole fruit.

4. Freeze fruit juice in an ice-cube tray, and use the frozen cubes to flavor your water, club soda, or seltzer water.

5. Drink fruit juice from designated "juice" glasses—they normally hold six ounces.

✔ *How's It Going?*
Are you weighing yourself weekly? If you're avoiding the scale, are your clothes fitting looser?

COFFEE AND TEA DRINKS: TO SAVE CALORIES, SCALE DOWN AND SIMPLIFY

If you expected me to tell you that you have to give up your one or two cups of coffee in the morning, relax. That small amount will get you going safely. More than that (from four to seven cups a day, or 500 to 600 milligrams of caffeine) can cause unpleasant side effects in many people, including sleeplessness, headaches, and anxiety.

What I do suggest is that you keep an eye on your consumption of "fancy" coffee or tea drinks, the kind often topped with syrup and whipped cream. If you're not careful, their added sugar and calories can cause an unpleasant side effect, too: weight gain.

Be brave and check the coffee chain's website or in-store nutrition information to find out the calorie count for brand coffee or tea drinks. Then log it in your journal, along with the serving size. Despite the hefty amount of calories these beverages can contain, there are often "skinnier" alternatives on the menu—give them a try. Also, reduce your serving size from grande or vente to tall—you'll reduce the calories you take in, too.

Even regular coffee or tea from your own pot or kettle can pack a surprising amount of calories if you have a heavy hand with sugar, half and half, or powdered creamer. If you add honey to your tea or coffee (some people do), you're adding sugar—64 calories per tablespoon, which should be logged in your food journal.

When it comes to coffee and tea drinks, my recommendation is to go retro. Have a good old-fashioned cup of Joe, black or with a touch of milk and one tablespoon of sugar or artificial sweetener, or a nice cup of tea with a squeeze of lemon or low-fat milk. Order iced coffee or iced tea unsweetened, and add your own low-fat milk and/or a small amount of sugar or artificial sweetener.

Most of the coffee excuses I hear have to do with sweeteners. Does either of these sound familiar?

I like my coffee really sweet.

Small Change Solution: One packet of regular sugar contains just 11 calories, so it's fine to add up to four packets—that's less than 50 calories. However, if you consume many cups of coffee per day and you use more than four packets at a time, switch to an artificial or alternative 0-calorie sweetener. The bottom line: The calories in your cup of coffee should not equal those in a piece of chocolate cake.

I love my cappuccino or latte [or other coffee-shop beverage]. I don't want to give it up.

Small Change Solution: You don't have to totally give up that drink, but you'll need to splurge with moderation if you want to reach your weight goal. Limit yourself to one tall (or grande, max) coffee-house beverage per day, and order it with nonfat milk or with a soy beverage. Soy has a naturally sweet flavor.

Small Change Coffee and Tea Drink Tips

1. Order lattes and cappuccinos with nonfat milk and unsweetened, one per day.

2. Use no more than four sugar packets daily and try adding cinnamon to your drink for some natural sweetness.

3. Switch down from vente to grande, grande to tall.

4. Request sugar-free syrups if ordering a "fancy" drink.

5. Skip the whipped cream on top of coffee drinks, which adds calories and fat.

ALCOHOL: TO SLIM DOWN, DRINK SENSIBLY

Many of my patients expect me to tell them that they have to go on the wagon to lose weight. But you don't have to give up alcohol completely—just fit it into your lifestyle, so it doesn't derail your goals.

Alcohol contains a fair amount of calories. When a shot is combined with soda, juice, or a prepared mix, the calorie count can go much higher. What's more, alcohol can impair judgment—including food judgment. After a few drinks, dieters tend to forget their good intentions and make poor food choices. Their inhibition drops, and the next thing they know, they've ordered deep-fried mozzarella sticks or polished off a whole bowl of peanuts. Also, people with hangovers tend not to eat healthfully, so your next day could wind up being a repeat performance.

To enjoy a daily libation *and* lose weight, limit yourself to one glass of that perfect red wine or one pint of your favorite beer on tap. Or opt for a less-caloric drink. For example, swap that draft beer for light beer in a bottle, or if you typically enjoy rum and cola, order it with diet cola, and limit yourself to one. If you drink vodka and orange juice, select a drink made without juice. In fact, as a general rule, avoid drinks made with soda or juice, and limit frozen drinks, like piña coladas and daiquiris, to vacation *only*. Also, like any other drinks, alcoholic beverages need to make it into your food journal.

One more thing: Be honest with yourself about how much you drink. One five-ounce glass of wine a day can be healthy (red wine in moderation is linked to cardiovascular health, for instance), and one drink might be your pleasure at the end of a hard day. However, overdrinking or binge drinking on the weekends is neither. In fact, heavy drinking is associated with cardiovascular disease, certain cancers, and other chronic health problems.

If you don't drink, you don't need to start. But if you do, drink responsibly, so your driving—and diet—are safe.

Beverage	Calories per 1 fluid ounce (approximate)	Serving (in ounces)	Total calories (approximate)
Beer, regular	12	12	144
Beer, light	9	12	108
Wine, white	20	5	100
Wine, red	21	5	105
Wine, sweet dessert	47	3	141
Distilled spirits (80-proof gin, rum, vodka, whiskey)	64	1.5	96

There's no reason to avoid alcohol completely when you're trying to lose weight. But if you choose to have a cocktail, it's important to avoid the excuses and pitfalls below.

I like only frozen margaritas [or other high-calorie cocktails].

Small Change Solution: If you drink them on occasion, like when away on vacation, enjoy! But if it's your usual cocktail, you need to reassess. A Long Island Iced Tea—which contains equal parts vodka, tequila, rum, gin, and triple sec, 1½ parts sweet-and-sour mix, and a splash of Coke—packs almost 800 calories! A Piña Colada (3 ounces light rum and 3 tablespoons each of milk and crushed pineapple) packs almost 700 calories, while a White Russian (2 ounces vodka and 1.5 ounces each of coffee liqueur and heavy cream) weighs in at 425 calories. The choice is yours: Downsize the calories in your cocktail or upsize your clothing.

I always go out after work with my coworkers. I'll feel left out if I don't drink.

Small Change Solution: Sure, you can have a drink—one, though, not five. Also, stick to lower-calorie drinks, such as vodka and club soda, rum and diet cola, light beer, or white wine. Or order a sparkling water with lime, which looks like a cocktail but sure doesn't have the calories of one.

Small Change Alcoholic Beverage Tips

1. Switch from regular beer to light beer.

2. If your drink of choice is made with tonic, switch to club soda instead; if it's made with cola, order it with diet soda.

3. Order a margarita on the rocks rather than a frozen margarita.

4. Alternate between your alcoholic beverage of choice and a glass of seltzer or water.

5. Before you go out for a drink, have a snack, like a piece of string cheese with fruit, a cup of nonfat yogurt and a piece of fruit, or a slice of cheese with several whole-grain crackers. It will help you drink less.

ARE YOU READY TO MOVE ON?

This Small Change can be a challenging one—so many people drink more calories than they think! The good news is, once you're aware of how sugar-sweetened beverages can impact your weight, it's tough to unlearn that lesson—and easier to slim down what you drink and to enjoy low- or zero-calorie alternatives. Take the Small Change Success Test below to see if you are ready to move on to the next Small Change.

Small Change Success Test

1. Are you drinking eight cups of water a day?

2. Have you swapped regular sweetened soda for diet soda, seltzer water, or club soda?

3. Have you switched from whole milk to 1 percent low-fat or nonfat milk?

4. If you drink fruit drinks, is your juice 100 percent fruit juice, and are you drinking just eight ounces a day?

5. Have you limited, or cut out, "fancy" sugar-sweetened coffee drinks and are you drinking regular coffee with low-fat milk and less sugar?

6. If you drink alcohol, have you limited your intake to one to two 5-ounce glasses of wine or 12-ounce beers or one cocktail a day?

If you answered yes to only four of the items on this chapter's Small Change Success Test, keep striving toward healthier changes, I know you can do it.

If you've answered yes to five questions, congratulations. It's time to tackle another Small Change!

Give Your Carbs a Makeover

Many of my patients come to me with a bad case of "carb phobia"—a fear of carbohydrates stemming from the belief that carbs make you fat. Time and again, I listened to them say things like, "I don't eat bread," or, "Rice, pasta, and potatoes are bad for you."

Guess what—they're not. So why do so many people still believe that carbohydrates cause weight gain? Part of the reason: They forget about the importance of portion control. When most people think carbs, they think *big*: big plates of pasta or huge slices of Chicago-style pizza—minus the veggies, of course. They don't see carbs as part of the healthy plate, but the entire plate.

They also forget that many carbohydrates are actually good for you—apples and grapes, broccoli and potatoes (yes, potatoes!), brown rice and oatmeal, to name a few. These foods contain vitamins and other nutrients that protect your health as well as fiber, which helps manage your appetite so that you're less likely to overeat.

And even though the carbs are the body's prime source of energy, many still avoid or severely limit their carbs. However, eliminating an entire food group from your diet doesn't get you slim, especially if you happen to love that food group—and most people, myself included, love carbohydrates. Because if you love them and don't eat them, eventually you will feel deprived and may even abandon your healthy goals. Bagels and pasta are two of my favorite foods. I eat them, my patients eat them, and you can, too.

If you have carb phobia, it's time to face it so you can enjoy carbohydrates again without guilt. This Small Change will help you do just that—while you lose weight.

To overcome your fear of carbs, you need to know the truth about them, which is this: Eating carbohydrates doesn't make you fat. Eating *too many* of the *wrong types* of carbohydrates makes you fat. So when you eat them, there are only three questions you need to consider:

- **How much?** We're talking about portion control here.

- *What type?* More often than not, you want to choose carbs that are high in fiber.

- *Which "extras"?* The spreads on your bread and bagels, the sauce on your pasta, the topping on your potatoes . . . low-fat is the way to go.

EAT MORE (FIBER), WEIGH LESS

Let's take another look at the healthy plate from Small Change 2. Notice that there is a spot for carbohydrates and it is only one-quarter of the plate.

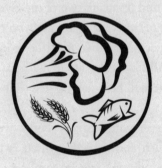

I tell my patients that before they fill that spot on their plate, they should ask themselves two questions:

1. Is my carb of choice high in fiber?

2. Am I watching my serving size?

If both answers are yes, you've made a smart choice for your health and your weight. The American Dietetic Association (ADA) recommends that an adult consume 25 to 35 grams of dietary fiber per day. The typical American gets just half that amount—roughly 10 to 15 grams a day.

Your body breaks down dietary fats, proteins, and carbohydrates. Dietary fiber, however—which comes only from plant foods—passes through your digestive system virtually intact. A diet rich in this indigestible stuff does more than keep you regular. A high-fiber diet also helps stabilize blood sugar, which helps control diabetes and lowers "bad" LDL cholesterol, reducing the risk of heart disease.

A high-fiber diet can also help you lose weight. You're more likely to not overeat. High-fiber foods have a low energy density, which means that you can have a larger portion with a lower number of calories.

Still, a calorie is a calorie. Eat calories in excess of what your body can burn, even in the form of high-fiber foods, and you'll gain weight. That means you need to watch your serving sizes. Following are some high-fiber choices that deserve that spot on your plate, along with how much of them is considered one serving:

- Barley: ½ cup cooked

- Breakfast cereal, high fiber: ¾ cup (average serving)

- Brown rice: ½ cup cooked

- Buckwheat: ½ cup cooked

- Legumes: (chickpeas, black beans, northern beans, kidney beans, etc.): ½ cup

- Oats: ½ cup dry

- Quinoa: ½ cup cooked

- Whole-wheat bread: 1 slice

- Whole-wheat couscous: ½ cup cooked

- Whole-wheat pasta: ½ cup cooked

- Wheatberries: ¼ cup dry

The bottom line is, to lose weight, you want to give your carbs a high-fiber makeover. And trust me, a high-fiber diet will look great on you.

Your Small Change Plan

1. Reduce your serving sizes.

2. Increase fiber at breakfast.

3. Brown your bread.

4. Fix your pasta.

5. Redo your rice.

6. Slim your potatoes.

THE WHOLE-GRAIN/FIBER CONNECTION

Some patients have asked me if *high fiber* and *whole grain* mean the same thing. Well, no—but where you find one, you find the other.

Grains are the seeds of plants. Fiber is a part of grains—whole grains, at least. Before they are processed, all grains have three components: the bran (where most of the fiber is), the germ (where most of the nutrients are), and the endosperm (which makes up the bulk of the seed).

Every grain starts out as a whole grain. But when a grain is refined, its bran and the germ are stripped away, leaving only the endosperm. Without the fiber and nutrient-dense bran and germ, about 25 percent of a grain's protein and more than fifteen key nutrients are lost.

Yes, vitamins and minerals are added back into refined grains after they are milled. (Manufacturers are even adding fiber to products made with refined grains now.) However, refined grains don't provide these nutrients naturally, and when it comes to food, natural is always better.

The percentage of fiber in a whole grain varies greatly, and it's fiber that fills you up so that you eat less but leave the table satisfied.

SERVE YOURSELF LESS, LOSE MORE WEIGHT

There's no way around it—when you reduce your serving sizes, you eat less. But if you use the Healthy Plate method, downsizing servings of protein and starchy carbohydrates as you upsize servings of fiber-rich carbs like vegetables and fruit, you won't leave the table hungry.

When you first tackle this small step, don't stress about the fiber content of the carbohydrates you put on your plate. It's enough to know that fiber fills you up. Before long, you'll automatically load your plate with it. Focus on serving size first.

I tell my patients to measure out some of their favorite carbohydrate foods onto a plate or bowl with a measuring cup so they can see what ½ cup of rice or ¾ cup of breakfast cereal actually looks like. After a week of measuring out servings, they can try to eyeball that same amount. Here are some examples of eyeballing to help you visualize what a serving size should look like:

One serving of bread = 1 slice of bread = the size of a CD case. You would think that one serving of bread, from a commercial loaf, would be one slice. Not necessarily. Along with most foods, loaves of sandwich bread have expanded in size, so one slice of a big, heavy loaf may be 1.5 or even 2 servings. Check the Nutrition Facts label on the brand you buy. You may be shocked to see that two slices amounts to three or even four servings of bread, rather than two.

Many of my patients ask, "If I have bread at breakfast, can I have a sandwich at lunch?" Yes. But that bread is your serving of carbohydrates at your midday meal, other than the carbs in your fruit and veggie servings. And what most don't realize is it is okay to have two servings (two slices of bread) if you are eating correct serving sizes.

By the way, one serving of a bagel is *not* one bagel, but half of it—the size of a hockey puck. Scoop out the center, too, since most bagels these days are very large.

One serving of cereal = ½ to ¾ cup = the amount that would fit in your cupped hands. The serving size often depends on the density of the cereal. If it's very dense, like granola, the serving size is smaller. So before you pour, check that label, then measure out one serving.

One serving of cooked pasta, rice, or other grain = ½ cup = the size of half a tennis ball. I tell my patients that they can have ½ cup cooked pasta, rice, or other grain with a meal—and if they have any, no bread. If you're used to heaping servings of pasta or grains, it's okay to scale down gradually. For example, if you currently eat 2 cups of rice at dinner, scale back to 1 cup, then ⅔ cup, and finally to ½ cup. But for some of my patients, those who are tall and/or active, I tell them they may be able to stop at 1 cup and still lose weight.

Not surprisingly, none of my patients like being told to reduce their serving sizes. Here are a few of the more common excuses:

I like my sandwiches in pita breads or wraps, not sliced bread.

Small Change Solution: Many of my patients prefer specialty breads too, especially wraps. As long as the brand you choose is made with whole wheat or whole grain, and is not ginormous, enjoy! Just choose a brand that contains 200 calories or fewer per serving. Take a look at "Sandwiches: Order Smart, Eat Smart" on page 112, too.

Do I have to give up crackers? I love my snack of cheese and crackers!

Small Change Solution: So do I! Whole-grain crackers or crispbreads and a slice of low-fat cheese make a tasty and satisfying snack. Just remember my mantra: Check the serving size on the Nutrition Facts label. Never eat crackers (or any other packaged food) straight from the box. If the serving size is five crackers, remove five, and then seal the box.

Small Changes Portion Size Tips

1. Prepare your plate in the kitchen, measuring out correct portions, rather than serve yourself from pots and dishes on the table.

2. Replace oversized or fluffy breads to save calories. Move from a whole bagel to a bialy or English muffin, from a sub, hoagie, or plain roll to sliced bread.

3. Use measuring cups to ensure correct serving size.

4. When you're comfortable with the measuring cups, start "eyeballing" portions.

5. Never eat out of a box or bag. Remove one portion, then close the bag.

INCREASE FIBER WITH BREAKFAST

There are good reasons to add fiber to breakfast. First, thanks to cereals and toast, it's easy to boost fiber in the morning, and when you eat healthfully in the morning, you set the tone for the entire day. Just as important, a fiber-full breakfast (and some more fiber in your midmorning snack) helps rein in your hunger until lunchtime.

Another bonus: Whatever you have for breakfast, there's a way to add fiber to it. Have a serving of fruit, opt for whole-grain toast instead of white, add veggies to your omelet, make pancakes and waffles with buckwheat instead of white flour. Or—and this is so easy—pour a bowl of high-fiber breakfast cereal that contains at least five grams of fiber per serving. (Oatmeal contains only four grams per serving, but it's so good for you that it's an exception to the rule.)

Five grams may sound like a lot, but many brands offer even more than that. Bran Buds, All-

Bran with Extra Fiber, and Fiber One contain 13, 13, and 14 grams of fiber per serving, respectively. If you don't like those, hit the cereal aisle and read those Nutrition Facts labels.

One thing to watch out for: added sugar. Even high-fiber cereals can pack a lot of it, which drives up the calories per serving. As a rule of thumb, the grams of fiber per serving in your cereal should be higher than its grams of sugar per serving. You can always add sweetness with fruit.

Once you find that high-fiber, lower-in-sugar brand, prepare to not be hungry for a while, as all that fiber keeps your hunger at bay. In a 2009 study, researchers in Toronto fed two groups of people breakfast. The first group got a low-fiber breakfast cereal with 1 percent milk. The second group was given a high-fiber variety (which contained 28.5 grams of fiber per serving), again with 1 percent milk. Three hours after that meal, the researchers gave both groups pizza, and told them to eat until they felt comfortably full. Compared to the group who'd eaten the low-fiber cereal at breakfast, those who'd eaten the high-fiber cereal consumed fewer calories from breakfast and lunch combined. They also said they felt more satisfied.

As important as it is to add fiber to breakfast, always pair your carbs with a serving of protein—

low-fat milk with your cereal, scrambled egg whites with your high-fiber pancakes, low-fat cottage cheese with your oatmeal, fruit, or toast. Remember, protein is part of a healthy plate, too—and without it in your morning meal, you are more likely to be starved two hours after you eat breakfast.

If you don't currently eat a fiber-rich breakfast, you probably have your reasons, like those below. My response: There are more good reasons to start.

I don't love the taste of high-fiber cereal . . . I prefer my sugar-coated brand.

Small Change Solution: One easy small change is to mix half a serving of the high-fiber variety with half a serving of your favorite brand. Every little bit of fiber helps keep hunger at bay. Eventually, try to wean yourself off the sugary stuff. Who knows? You might actually start to like your high-fiber brand.

I can't give up my favorite takeout breakfast sandwich on a croissant.

Small Change Solution: You might love it, but it's probably low in fiber and high in fat and calories. Switch your order to an egg, or scrambled egg whites (add some veggies if you like) and whole-wheat toast spread with a single pat of butter. Or make this sandwich yourself, at home. It's a healthy combo of fiber and protein. And who knows, it may become your new favorite.

I can't eat fiber because it makes me bloated and gassy.

Small Change Solution: That's probably because you don't eat that much of it, and your digestive system isn't used to it. Add fiber gradually to your diet, rather than 30 grams the first day. That gives the natural bacteria in your digestive system a chance to get used to the extra roughage. Make sure to drink enough fluid, too—it helps fiber pass through the digestive system more easily.

Small Change Fiber-for-Breakfast Tips

1. "Cut" your current high-sugar cereal with a low-sugar, high-fiber brand. Gradually reduce the amount of sugared cereal in your bowl until you are eating only the high-fiber brand.

2. To add extra fiber to your breakfast cereal, add 1 tablespoon of ground flaxseed.

3. Use quick-cooking oatmeal (not instant oatmeal, which can be high in sugar), which takes 2 minutes in the microwave. Sprinkle on cinnamon for sweetness.

4. As an alternative to oatmeal, try quinoa,
    now available in the grain section of most
    supermarkets. Stir in a dollop of low-fat
    yogurt and top with fruit.

5. For delicious, high-fiber pancakes and waffles,
    make them with buckwheat flour and sweeten
    with berries or sliced bananas. Watch your
    portions.

BROWN YOUR BREAD

When I meet patients for the first time, I ask
them what foods they love. Inevitably, bread is at
the top of the list. No surprise there—good bread
is one of the great pleasures of life. Still, there can
be too much of a good thing—and today's bread
isn't the nutritious loaf of a century ago—unless
it's made with whole grains.

Typically, high-fiber breads are made with unre-
fined grains—that is, they don't have the bran and
husk stripped away during its processing into flour.
(When those parts are removed, you have white
flour.) However, many commercial loaves sound
like they're healthy—but their names can fool you.
Often, those "7-grain," "multigrain," and "hearty"

breads contain mostly refined white flour and little or no fiber. The color of bread isn't always helpful either. Many dark breads only look hearty, thanks to artificial color or molasses.

To make sure your bread is bona fide whole grain, even if it looks to you like it is made with whole grains, check the Nutrition Facts label. It should say, "100 percent whole grain," or, "100 percent whole wheat." Don't be fooled by its appearance or these terms:

- *Whole grain:* If the label doesn't say "100 percent whole grain," it may have many grain blends. Words you don't want to see alongside "flour" include "bleached," "unbleached," "semolina," and "durum."

- *Made with whole grains:* The bread may contain *some* whole grains, but unless it's 100 percent, you won't reap the fiber or the potential health benefits.

- *Multigrain:* That means "more than one grain"—but are those grains whole or refined? You just don't know.

Now that you know how to identify whole-grain bread, enjoy it responsibly. These suggestions can help. *Sandwich bread:* Try to stick with sliced bread of a standard-sandwich size—leave the over-sized loaves on the shelf. My rule of thumb: per slice, 100 calories, max, and 3 grams of fiber, minimum.

Pita bread and wraps: Check the serving size on the Nutrition Facts label. One large wrap may count as two servings.

Bagels: Scoop out the inside and opt for low-fat fillings and spreads.

Specialty breads and rolls: French or Italian bread, or hard or soft rolls, shouldn't be an everyday choice—they're typically high in calories but light on fiber.

What about croissants, biscuits, and dinner rolls? Well, if you can find a whole-grain version with at least three grams of fiber, you can have it. But count it as your carb serving—have one, enjoy it, and stop.

Of all the excuses I hear, many concern beloved bread.

I like only white bread.

Small Change Solution: Have you tried whole-wheat bread? One of my patients, a self-described "picky eater," claimed to dislike it. But I persuaded her to swap her roll (every day, she ate a turkey sandwich on a roll for lunch) for whole-wheat bread. What do you know—she liked it. She's eaten turkey on whole wheat since and is eight pounds lighter. But if you can't switch now, try the white breads with added fiber—two slices have five grams. However, aim to switch to breads with naturally occurring fiber.

I love the fresh-baked bakery bread—it's all I eat.

Small Change Solution: No problem, if you buy real whole-wheat or whole-grain bread. Just ask the counterperson to slice your loaf into "sandwich slices" for you. Also, keep your loaf in the freezer and take out one serving at a time, so you won't be tempted to eat more of it than you want to.

I can't eat bread at all, because once I start I can't stop.

Small Change Solution: As with any trigger food, if you really can't eat it in moderation no matter how hard you try, avoid it. You don't need to eat bread. Simply get your fiber from high-fiber breakfast cereal, oatmeal and other whole grains, and fruit and veggies. You could also eat bread in sandwich form only—the portion is right there in front of you.

Small Change Bread Tips

1. Choose breads that contain a maximum of 100 calories and a minimum of 3 grams of fiber per serving.

2. Choose presliced bread over rolls.

3. If bread is part of your meal, skip other starches, such as rice, potatoes, and pasta.

4. Scoop out bread with a doughy inside.

5. Pass on the "bread basket" at restaurants.

SANDWICHES: ORDER SMART, EAT SMART

While specialty breads like Italian focaccia or *ciabatta,* French baguettes, and Italian bread are delicious, as are sandwiches made on them, they tend to be calorie dense and fiber light. But you can still enjoy them, if you eat smart. The following tips can help. While the guidelines address sandwiches, they work if you eat the bread by itself, too.

If you order a sandwich on bread with a doughy inside (including bagels, long steak or hoagie rolls, and plain hard or soft rolls), ask to have the inside scooped out before the filling is added. Scooped bagels are delicious with natural peanut butter and low-sugar jam, or a smear of light cream cheese and egg whites; for other breads, low-fat turkey and veggies, with mustard, is a smart and tasty choice.

Sandwiches that come on any bread other than standard sliced bread are typically huge, and definitely more than one serving. If you order a sandwich that looks like it would feed two or more people, eat half and wrap the other half to go.

Panini (hot, pressed sandwiches of Italian origin) tend to be large, too. Usually, half of a restaurant or deli panino would be a portion. Or make your own panini at home, with sliced whole-grain bread.

Stick with healthy fillings—lean deli meat like turkey or grilled chicken (more on lean meats in Small Change 6) and lots of veggies. Opt for low-fat cheese, if possible, or skip it altogether, and go easy on the mayo.

If your sandwich contains so much meat that you can't get your mouth around it, remove half and use it in another sandwich within the next day or so.

It's tough to know the fiber content of specialty bread, especially if you order it at a restaurant. If the restaurant offers whole-grain sliced bread, however, opt for it. It may contain some fiber and be closer to an appropriate portion.

FIX YOUR PASTA

I hate when people say that pasta is "bad for you." It's not pasta that makes you fat. What makes you fat is having an entire plate of it, on a plate as big as a bowling ball, with too much meat or cream sauce and no veggies or lean protein. My point: To protect your arteries and waistline, don't build a meal around pasta. Eat pasta as *part of your meal*. There's a huge difference.

When you include pasta with your meal, it takes up a quarter of your plate, and amounts to about 1 cup. Build that cup with lean protein and veggies, and you get the pasta you crave, and the added fiber and protein will help fill you up.

So if you are in the mood for pasta, serve yourself a cup (preferably the whole-wheat variety for the fiber). Then add 1 cup of veggies—asparagus, broccoli, or spinach are yummy—and 4 ounces of lean protein, such as grilled chicken or shrimp (if you want a vegetarian meal, use ½ cup of beans instead). For sauce, use ½ cup of a plain marinara without added sugar or other sweeteners. Or make your own sauce with chunks of fresh tomato, mushrooms, zucchini, or eggplant—the veggies offer fiber as well as other nutrients. Top your sauce with 1 tablespoon of grated Parmesan.

One of my patients, Stephanie, twenty-four, lost

her fifteen extra pounds *and* ate pasta, one of her favorite foods. She'd associated carbs with gaining weight—low-carb diets had scared her off them. "Now I don't run away from a pasta meal—as long as I eat the whole-wheat kind, with a serving of protein and tons of veggies," she said. She's kept off those fifteen pounds for more than a year.

After all I've told you, you shouldn't have any excuses about pasta. But in case you do . . .

I don't like the taste of whole-wheat pasta.

Small Change Solution: Remember the cereal trick? It works with pasta, too. Mix half regular pasta and half the whole-wheat variety for a while, and gradually switch to whole wheat entirely. Try different brands of whole-wheat pasta, too, because they don't all taste the same. While whole-wheat pasta is an acquired taste, if you never acquire a taste for it, don't worry. If you limit yourself to the one-cup maximum, you're still ahead of the game.

But I love the pasta at my favorite Italian place.

Small Change Solution: So have it—just build your meal around the healthy plate. You have two options. First, you can order a grilled fish or chicken entrée with a half order of pasta (choose a lighter sauce, like meatless marinara or olive oil and garlic). Or, if you want pasta as an entrée, eat one cup of it (remember, that's about the size of a tennis ball) or ask for a half order if available. Then build your meal with a side of veggies, so you don't leave the table hungry. (More on dining out in Small Change 9.)

Regardless of which option you choose, skip the bread—you're having pasta. If your favorite place won't accommodate a half order of pasta (most restaurants will), buy the full order and ask that half be put in a "to go" box rather than on your plate.

Pasta is such a quick, inexpensive meal, I can't afford not to eat it!

Small Change Solution: Well, it is inexpensive, and you can eat it. Just keep to the simple "formula" of pasta, protein, and veggies: Open a jar of tomato sauce, microwave a bag of veggies, throw in half a can of beans, top with a bit of Parmesan, and you have a quick, inexpensive, and *healthy* meal.

Small Change Pasta Tips

1. Watch your portion of pasta—just a quarter of the plate.

2. Build your pasta *meal* with veggies and lean protein, not more pasta.

---

3. When you order pasta in a restaurant, request a half order.

4. Switch to whole-wheat pasta—its fiber will help fill you up.

5. When you have pasta, pass on the bread.

YES, YOU CAN EAT PIZZA

Relieved? I thought you would be. You don't even have to order it with a whole-wheat crust (which is very hard to find, anyway). To enjoy pizza and still lose weight, it's all about portion and toppings.

With pizza, there's really no standard serving size; one slice contains about 300 calories, which means one slice fits into a balanced diet, even when you're eating healthy. One slice, not two, four, or a whole pie.

Use pizza as an opportunity to add fiber-rich veggies to your diet. They're high in nutrients and flavor. Pass on the meats. Sausage, pepperoni, or other meats add only fat and calories to your healthy slice. Order it with veggies, request a thin crust, and ask for more sauce and half the cheese. You truly won't miss it. If you have the option of ordering a whole-wheat crust, take it.

A "personal pizza" is okay on occasion, but if you

order one, skip the meats and order it with veggies. And enjoy a side salad with your slice, or rare individual pie, to help fill you up.

✔ **How's It Going?**

If you've made any poor food choices, were you able to get immediately back on track?

REDO YOUR RICE

Notice I didn't say, "Give up your rice." That's because rice isn't the problem. It's the quantity that most people eat, as well as the butter, cheese, or other "extras" that are added to it. So make sure your rice serving takes up no more than a quarter of your plate, and use low-fat, low-calorie flavorings (i.e., herbs and spices). Hot sauce is great, as is a teaspoon or two of Parmesan cheese. Or if cooking your rice in water is not flavorful for you, try cooking it in a low-sodium vegetable or fat-free chicken broth.

Also, choose brown rice as often as you can. It's not that white rice is bad, but brown rice is more nutritious and well worth the few extra minutes of cooking time. And honestly, once you make the switch, you'll realize that it's far more flavorful.

Don't limit yourself to rice either. Because whole

grains contain the most fiber and nutrients, they should always be your first choice. Research shows that they help reduce the risk of heart disease and diabetes. Experiment with some of the whole grains below.

- Amaranth
- Barley
- Brown rice
- Buckwheat
- Bulgur wheat
- Kamut
- Millet
- Oats
- Quinoa
- Rye
- Wheat
- Whole-wheat couscous
- Wild rice

With all that brown rice and other whole grains have going for them, it's hard to come up with excuses not to eat them. Still, people try.

Brown rice takes too long to make.

Small Change Solution: Not anymore—you can find quick-cooking varieties at the supermarket. Chinese restaurants offer brown rice, too, so if you're pressed for time, pick up a small container at your local Chinese place. Just make sure not to eat the entire container.

I love rice and beans, and thought it was good for me, especially the beans, right?

Small Change Solution: Rice and beans can be a very nutritious dish, as long as you watch the portion. Beans are an excellent source of fiber, as long as they're prepared without a lot of fat (sausage or other pork, coconut milk, or loads of cheese). So, if you make this dish yourself, prepare it without fatty ingredients, or at least pare them down a lot. You might start by adding peppers, onions, tomatoes, and garlic to boost flavor and nutrients. Also experiment with using brown rice instead of white. Then, do a portion check—a quarter of your plate for "rice," and that includes the beans (1 cup total).

Don't ask me to give up my sushi rolls!

Small Change Solution: I don't ask anyone to give up anything, as long as they can fit it into their balanced diet and watch their portion sizes. To lose weight and still enjoy your sushi, I recommend that you limit yourself to two rolls, and add some edamame (soy beans) and a side salad. (And if you can get sushi made with brown rice, go for it.)

Small Change Rice and Grains Tips

1. If it looks like too much, it is. Stick to a ½-cup serving.

2. Cook grains in water or low-sodium and fat-free veggie broth or chicken broth rather than oil and butter.

3. Be adventurous. If you like white rice, try brown. Or try some of the more exotic whole grains.

4. Make extra grains for tomorrow night's dinner.

5. If you enjoy rice with your meal, pass on the bread. (This is so important, it bears repeating.)

SLIM YOUR POTATOES

Packed with fiber (especially the skin) and potassium, potatoes are good for you. The problem: Most people can't leave well enough alone. They pile an enormous baked potato with butter and sour cream, or cheese and bacon bits. Or eat huge servings of French fries, sometimes with melted cheese. Or load mashed potatoes with too much butter, whole milk, or cream. From scalloped potatoes to hash browns, "loaded" baked potatoes to potato chips, we've turned this healthy food into a disaster.

That's not to say you can never eat potatoes this way again. (Hey, I love French fries, too!) But you can't eat them every day. If you watch your portions and can pare down the fatty toppings and add-ins, you can still enjoy your potatoes as you pare down your weight. The magic words are *portion* and *preparation*.

First, let's tackle serving size. One serving of baked potato (white or sweet), is the size of a computer mouse, while a serving of mashed potatoes is ½ cup. One serving of French fries is two to three ounces (in restaurants, that's roughly the size of a "small" bag). And guess what? Those amounts take up a quarter of your plate.

Now, for preparation. An across-the-board recommendation: Eat the skin of your potato—it contains most of the fiber. If you make fries, cut them into wedges with the skin on. If you make mashed potatoes, don't peel them first. And don't leave the skin of your baked potato on your plate—it can help fill you up, and it's delicious, especially when it's been baked to a crisp.

Baked potato: You can top your potato with one pat of butter (45 calories), but hold the bacon bits and melted cheese. Healthy alternatives include 2 tablespoons low-fat sour cream, ¼ cup low-fat cottage cheese, salsa, mustard, or even hummus (my personal favorite is black-bean hummus).

Mashed potatoes: Swap the butter, whole milk, cream, cheese, and regular sour cream for low-fat or nonfat milk and nonfat sour cream. Top your serving with a sprinkle of Parmesan.

Or make smashed potatoes, using tiny red new potatoes: Boil the potatoes, leaving the skin on for the fiber. Smash them with mustard or add a little olive oil and top with Parmesan.

French fries: I know fast-food fries are tasty, but baked fries are, too. Coat a baking pan with cooking spray. Slice a whole potato into thin strips, place the strips on the pan, spritz with 1 tablespoon of olive oil and rosemary, toss to coat. Bake at 450 degrees for about 45 minutes, turning at least once for even browning.

Just as with bread, people offer many reasons why they can't give up potatoes.

My spouse supersizes his fries, and I can't resist them. In fact, I end up eating half of them!

Small Change Solution: I always say it's better to

eat off someone else's plate than your own—you're less likely to overeat. But if he's supersizing, and you're eating half, consider getting a small fries for yourself—you'll actually eat fewer fries! This is an occasional treat, not an everyday occurrence. Or, try to convince your spouse to swap his fries for a side salad with low-fat dressing. After all, his health and waistline are important, too.

I'd love to eat a potato, but the ones in the store are huge!

Small Change Solution: It does seem like potatoes have supersized, along with virtually every other food. But the solution is simple: If you can't buy a small potato, buy a larger one, slice it in half before you prepare it, and enjoy. Or, if you're sure you won't succumb to temptation, cook it all, and save the other half for tomorrow night's dinner.

There's no way I can give up potato chips.

Small Change Solution: I'm not opposed to chips. Just eat one serving—usually one ounce. Also, count them as your carb at lunch or dinner (or as your snack). So enjoy them at lunch with a salad or half a sandwich (one slice of bread), and skip other carbohydrate foods if you eat them at dinner. If you eat them as a snack, pair them with protein, like a slice of cheese. You might also try baked chips, again eating just one serving.

Small Change Potato Tips

1. Watch your portions—measure out ½ cup of mashed potatoes and choose a small baked potato.

2. Top baked potatoes with low-fat toppings.

3. Swap fried potatoes for baked fries.

4. Prepare mashed potatoes with nonfat milk and low-fat sour cream.

5. If you really want hash browns with your eggs, skip the toast.

ARE YOU READY TO MOVE ON?

Hopefully, your carb phobia is history. With a renewed respect for serving size, you've learned how to fit all your favorites—bread, potatoes, pasta, bagels, maybe even pizza—into a healthier, more fiber-full diet. Not so scary, when you take it one step at a time.

Take the Small Change Success Test on the next page to see if you are ready to move on to the next Small Change.

Small Change Success Test

1. Have you increased your intake of fiber at breakfast?

2. Have you reduced your serving sizes of bread and other carbohydrate foods?

3. Did you swap your white sandwich bread for fiber-rich whole-wheat or other whole-grain bread?

4. Do you make pasta a part of your plate, instead of the whole plate?

5. Are you sticking to ½ cup of brown rice or other whole grain?

6. Have you slimmed your potatoes?

If you answered yes to only four of the items on this chapter's Small Change Success Test, go back to the plan and keep plugging away at the Small Changes that challenge you, one at a time. It may take you a while to work your way through the list, but if my patients can do it, so can you!

If you've answered yes to five questions, congratulations. It's time to tackle another Small Change!

▼▲▼▲▼▲▼▲▼

Go Easy on the "Extras" and Make Savory Swaps for Old Standbys

Some of the highest-fat, highest-calorie foods we eat aren't foods at all. They're "extras"—items we put *on* food to add flavor. These include butter, sour cream, mayonnaise, gravy, and salad dressings, as well as pasta sauces (white, creamy sauces are the worst offenders) and various spreads and toppings.

Gina, forty-nine, loved her morning bagel slathered with butter, her lunchtime tuna fish loaded up with mayonnaise, and her homemade spaghetti Bolognese—a meat sauce packed with ground beef—for dinner. However, she did not love that she weighed 263 pounds. When I met with her, I told her straight: Her love of high-fat "extras" like butter and mayonnaise was derailing her attempts to lose weight.

But Gina's will to lose weight was stronger than her love for butter. With my help, she began to swap high-fat dressings, spreads, and sauces for low-fat alternatives. Her Bolognese sauce received the first makeover. Instead of ground beef, she used veggie crumbles made with soy protein, which are only 70 calories per serving. "I didn't taste the difference," she said. Gina also traded in her morning buttered bagel for an egg-white sandwich. Instead of using full-fat cheese, she substituted a wedge of low-fat cheese flavored with garlic or onion, which added a lot of flavor for only 35 calories.

Thirteen months later, Gina was fifty-six pounds lighter.

Remember, to lose a pound a week, you need to consume 500 fewer calories a day. If you give up two tablespoons of butter on your breakfast toast, one tablespoon of mayo and a slice of cheese in your lunchtime sandwich, and a dollop of sour cream on your baked potato at dinner, you've trimmed just about that much without eating less food!

Of course, few of us want to eat these foods "naked"—and fortunately, we don't have to. Use low-fat versions of sour cream, mayo, cheese, and dips, and punch up flavor with herbs, spices, and low-fat condiments. If you like to cook, swap out high-fat ingredients like butter, oil, and mayo for their low-fat counterparts.

It's not easy to give up butter, homemade gravy, your favorite blue-cheese dressing, or *alfredo* sauce on your pasta. I've had clients who find it difficult to give up regular mayonnaise! But rather than focus on deprivation, keep your eyes on the prize: a slimmer, healthier you. I promise that you haven't been doomed to a life of flavorless food. If you open your mind (and mouth) to the alternatives, you'll find that you can give up fat without giving up flavor.

Your Small Change Plan

1. Ask for dressing, sauce, and gravy on the side.

2. Swap high-fat salad dressings for low-fat alternatives.

3. Slim your sauces.

4. Defat your spreads and toppings.

5. Use veggies as an "extra."

JUST SAY, "ON THE SIDE"

Remember the restaurant scenes in *When Harry Met Sally* where Sally requests everything from salad dressing to the ice cream for her pie à la mode "on the side"?

I can relate. When I was dating my husband and placed my order at a restaurant, he'd inevitably ask, afterward, "Can't you just eat a meal the way they make it?" I'd reply, "Why do I have to? I know what's best for me." (He married me anyway—and orders his dressing on the side now, too.)

My point: As long as you're polite, it's okay to be a Sally, because when you learn to say "on the side," you get the best of both worlds. You get to enjoy your favorite gravy, sour cream, salad dressing, butter, or hollandaise sauce. You just won't add an extra 200 or more calories to your meal.

This is a simple small change: Order any sauce, dressing, or gravy, as well as butter and sour cream, on the side. Often, you'll be given an amount that could serve a family of four, but serve yourself no more than two tablespoons. If you've requested butter on the side, have one pat.

The "on the side" strategy works nicely for my patients, and for me. I get to have the yummy balsamic vinaigrette on my salad, so I never feel deprived. Once you make this small change, you, too, may be surprised to find that two tablespoons satisfy you just fine.

This small step is so doable that my patients don't have a lot of objections. That said, here are the most common self-created roadblocks:

I can't eat [whatever] without [whatever].

Small Change Solution: Is it that you *can't* eat a baked potato without both butter and sour cream, or a salad without a ladle of blue-cheese dressing, or you *won't*? The point is moot, because you don't have to give up anything. You just have to get used to using less of it. There's a big difference.

It embarrasses me to make special requests.

Small Change Solution: It may feel that way, but only because you're not used to it. You're not making a fuss. Really. Servers hear special requests, including "on the side, please," all the time, and cooks are used to accommodating them. (I even request "on the side" in other countries, and haven't been turned down yet!) As long as you ask politely, you're no bother. Your reward for your newfound assertiveness? A slimmer you.

Small Change "On the Side" Tips

1. Learn to say, "on the side, please."

2. When you order toast, ask for butter on the side. You'll use less than if the kitchen butters it.

3. Order sandwiches without mayo, tartar sauce, or "special sauces." Ask for packets instead, then use a small amount.

4. Dip your fork into the sauce, then spear the food.

5. If your "on the side" request yields a large amount of dressing, gravy, or sauce, use two tablespoons *only*.

DEFAT YOUR SALAD DRESSINGS

A salad can be your best friend or worst enemy—it comes down to the kind of dressing you choose, and how much you use. Fortunately, it's not hard to turn around a salad disaster.

There are two basic types of dressings. The *creamy* kind (Thousand Island, Caesar, Russian, blue cheese, creamy Italian) has a base of high-fat ingredients like mayonnaise, sour cream, butter-milk, or heavy cream. The *oil and vinegar* type (balsamic vinaigrette, Italian) has a base of vegetable oil—olive, canola, and so forth.

If you buy bottled dressing, read the Nutrition Facts label closely before you choose a brand. Fat-free and low-fat dressings can be packed with sugar and other sweeteners, which will raise their calorie count, and some regular brands are high in unhealthy saturated fats. A healthier choice in bottled dressings is an oil-based brand made with canola or olive oil. You'll get the healthy monounsaturated fat and, in the case of canola oil, omega-3 fatty acids. While not etched in stone, a good guideline is to choose a brand that contains, per serving, no more than 40 calories, 6 grams of fat, and 1 gram of saturated fat.

Once you've found your dressing, pay attention to the amount you use. Note the serving size information on the Nutrition Facts label (in most cases, two tablespoons). If you regularly eat salad at work, keep a second bottle in the office. This way, you'll know exactly what your dressing contains, and you won't have to guess as you stand at the local salad bar.

If you have time, homemade dressings can be just as tasty—or tastier—than bottled varieties, and you have control over the ingredients. The key:

Reduce the oils and other fats, and pump up ingredients that add flavor.

You can even make your own creamy dressings with low-fat mayo, nonfat milk, low-fat buttermilk, and low-fat cottage cheese (which makes a good base for a blue-cheese dressing). If you prefer oil-based dressings, experiment with different types of oils. Extra-virgin olive oil and canola oil are excellent choices. So are flax and walnut. These specialty oils' subtle flavors can complement your veggies. Add Dijon mustard to vinaigrettes, or horseradish to creamy dressings. Experiment with herbs and spices, too. Use fresh herbs, if you can—their flavor is more intense than dried—and grind your own pepper and other spices.

As with bottled dressings, watch your serving size of homemade varieties. Stick to two tablespoons, so you won't rack up the calories. (I know you're using two tablespoons of high-fat dressings, too, but it's my hope that in time, you'll "graduate" to one that's lower in fat.)

Many people prefer a simple oil-and-vinegar dressing, my patients included. But I found that some of them used more oil than they needed. This tip helped them (I use it myself) and it can help you: Buy a plant mister, wash and dry it, then add your favorite oil. When you're ready for your salad, give your greens a quick spritz of oil (spray up to four times), and then add vinegar. If you feel you need extra flavor, top your salad with a tablespoon of Parmesan or feta cheese. You'll be surprised at how little oil a salad really needs.

Ladling on the dressing is more of a bad habit than a conscious decision. Even so, my patients have a few "reasons" for why they shouldn't have to stop doing so:

I don't like low-fat or fat-free dressings. To enjoy my salad, which I know I must eat, I need a lot of dressing.

Small Change Solution: You can't have everything, so choose quantity or taste. I suggest that you enjoy two tablespoons of the full-fat version, and add extra balsamic vinegar so your salad is more covered with dressing. Many of my clients depend on this trick.

I know I shouldn't have Caesar salad but I really enjoy it when I am out for dinner and I don't want to give it up.

Small Change Solution: You don't have to give up anything. Just enjoy it once a week. If you want it more often, make your own low-fat Caesar dressing at home, or order the dressing on the side.

Small Change Defat-Your-Dressing Tips

1. Opt for vinaigrettes more often than creamy dressings.

2. If you buy bottled dressing, watch for saturated fat and calories per serving.

3. Make over creamy dressings with low-fat or nonfat mayo, milk or buttermilk, and cottage cheese.

4. To reduce the amount of oil you use, put oil in a plant mister and spritz it on your salad.

5. To kick up the flavor of a plain oil-and-vinegar dressing, add your favorite mustard or horseradish.

SLIM YOUR SAUCES

My patients tend to worry too much about eating pasta, and not enough about the sauces they use to top it with. In general, the creamier the sauce, the more fat you put in your mouth and around your waistline.

While some people make their own pasta sauce, not everyone has the time or inclination, and they opt for the convenience of bottled or prepared sauces. If that sounds like you, check the Nutrition Facts label for serving size and calories and fat per serving. In general, red sauces such as marinara, pomodoro, tomato, or red clam are the lightest options. Creamy sauces like alfredo and alla vodka, as well as those with added meats like Bolognese, tend to pack tons of calories and saturated fat.

If you make your own pasta sauce, or want to try, you'll avoid the less-than-healthy additions that make their way into bottled sauces, including salt and sweeteners. You'll even be able to include a small amount of meat, if desired, as long as it's lean. (More on lean meats in Small Change 6.)

Since most of the fat in creamy pasta sauces comes from margarine or butter and milk, use skim milk, leave out the margarine or butter, and use vegetable broth instead of oil. Pasta primavera can be a light make-at-home choice, if you skip the cream and butter and make it as it was originally conceived—with lots of veggies, two teaspoons of olive oil, garlic, and a bit of fresh Parmesan.

When you're out to dinner, choose a pasta dish made with a red sauce, like those above, rather than heavy sauces made with butter, cream, cheese, meat, or too much oil. White clam sauce is fine, too. If you want pasta all'olio (oil), enjoy it as a side dish rather than as a main entrée. As a side dish (because it doesn't contain veggies or protein), pasta with garlic and oil can be a good choice. In fact, if you make it from home, it's the perfect opportunity to give your pasta a spritz from your oil bottle. Add flavor with garlic, red pepper flakes, a little minced parsley, and a sprinkle of Parmesan. Whatever pasta dish you order, stick to a 1-cup serving, and skip the bread.

Sauces aren't just for pasta, of course. They're also used to top meat, poultry, and fish, and every chef in every restaurant creates his or her own. (Even fast-food chains have their own proprietary special sauces, but it's no secret that they're full of fat and calories.) Rule of thumb: If they are creamy, they're not good for your waistline. Request them on the side and limit yourself to two tablespoons.

If you make a homemade meat sauce or gravy, use a fat separator to skim off the fat, or refrigerate until the fat rises to the top for easy removal.

I know it's difficult to give up heavy, creamy sauces, and I hear the same excuses for not doing it time and again:

I only like creamy pasta sauces, like alfredo or penne alla vodka.

Small Change Solution: Why give them up? Simply prepare lighter, waist-friendly versions at home. If it's just the creaminess you crave, stir two tablespoons of hummus into a red sauce. I've done this, and suggest it to my patients as well, who find it delicious. When you dine out, try a pasta dish with a lighter sauce. You may be surprised by how much you enjoy it.

I love my pesto sauce. It's green, so it's healthy, right?

Small Change Solution: Pesto is delicious, but mind-bogglingly high in fat. Besides basil, a traditional pesto contains ground pine nuts, olive oil, and Parmesan cheese, which is why a ¼ cup serving contains about 300 calories. I recommend that you enjoy it on occasion only. Or make a lower-fat, lower-calorie version at home—simply swap the olive oil for vegetable stock and use a smaller amount of pine nuts. Not exactly traditional, but you will save lots of calories.

Small Change Slim-Your-Sauces Tips

1. Choose red pasta sauces over white, creamy sauces.

2. Keep an eye on serving sizes—½ cup of red sauce; ¼ cup of white, creamy sauces.

3. Prepare homemade sauces with low-fat ingredients, like low-fat milk and vegetable broth.

4. Skim the fat from homemade gravy.

5. To give homemade red sauces a creamy texture, add two tablespoons of hummus.

Five Simple Strategies to Slim Your Pasta Sauce

- Top pasta with chopped vegetables and add ½ cup of your favorite bottled red sauce.

- Use fresh herbs—they're an easy way to add flavor. If you use fresh basil, add it at the last minute to maximize its fresh, delicate taste.

- For a quick, easy, nutrient-packed sauce, turn to your blender. Cook your favorite veggies, puree, add herbs and spices, and simmer. Pureed, roasted red peppers make a tasty sauce.

- Pair pasta with low-fat, fiber-rich legumes, such as beans and lentils, instead of fat-laden meat sauces.

- If you make your own pasta sauce, start with broths or vegetable purees as bases instead of cream and butter. If you must use fat, stick to small amounts of margarine with plant stanols or a quick spritz of olive oil or cooking spray.

✔ **How's It Going?**

Are you on track with your weight-loss goals? Are you still committed to your initial reason to lose weight?

LIGHTEN YOUR TOPPINGS AND SPREADS

What's toast without butter, or a baked potato without sour cream? That's what a lot of my patients ask when I recommend low-fat alternatives to these high-fat spreads and toppings. I tell them that they don't have to give them up—they just have to lighten them up.

While some of these alternatives may sound strange, taste before you judge. Many of my patients love the new flavors—you're bound to find at least a few you like.

Butter

If you can confine your serving to one to two pats, that's fine. But who can use so little, especially on toast? A better option: the newer vegetable spreads made with plant stanols. They taste delicious, come in a light version, and can help promote healthy cholesterol levels. Avoid any spread that contains hydrogenated oil. That's code for artery-clogging trans fats.

Cheese

Stick to low-fat cheese, or try flavoring with hummus instead. There are so many flavors to choose from that you likely won't even miss the cheese. Many of my patients loved to add cheese to their scrambled eggs. Now they add a few drops of Tabasco sauce or top with salsa, and the cheese is history.

Cream Cheese

Switch to the low-fat variety, or try "cream cheese" made from tofu. (I buy mine at the bagel store with chopped scallions added for extra flavor.) Believe it or not, many of my patients enjoy it. While tofu cream cheese contains fat, it's the healthy monounsaturated kind from soy beans. Read the Nutrition Facts label, though, to make sure the brand you buy is free of trans fats.

Many people like cream cheese with jelly or jam. Although these spreads aren't high in fat, they sure are high in calories. Opt for sugar-free versions that contain only 10 calories per tablespoon, or spread your toast or scooped bagel with two tablespoons of low-fat cottage or ricotta cheese. For sweetness add a sprinkle of cinnamon. Yum!

Mayonnaise

If you don't like the low-fat variety, use one tablespoon of regular mayo and one tablespoon of nonfat Greek yogurt, and aim to eventually make the switch to yogurt only. Or spread on some low-fat flavor with salsa, mustard, or hummus instead. (Tuna tastes great mixed with spicy brown mustard, for example.) I recommend spreading hummus on a sandwich just like you would mayo.

Sour Cream

Make dips with the low-fat variety or try low-fat yogurt. Top baked potatoes with a mixture of low-fat sour cream and hummus or low-fat cottage cheese—one tablespoon of each. It's delicious. Some of my patients top their baked spuds with horserad-ish, low-fat plain yogurt, or fat-free Greek yogurt, which is extrathick.

Think you "can't" give up your favorite high-fat spreads? So do many of my patients. Here are some common excuses—fortunately, I have answers for all of them.

Please don't tell me I have to give up ketchup.

Small Change Solution: I never tell anyone to give up a food they love. Besides, ketchup contains only 28 calories per 2-tablespoon serving. Buy the low-sodium variety if you monitor your salt intake, and stick to the recommended serving size.

I don't like steamed veggies unless I top them with butter.

Small Change Solution: You sound like my husband! And I would get upset that he was taking a nutritious food and making it fattening. I had to do an intervention. He now gets the buttery flavor he craves from a margarine made with plant stanols, which can be healthy and lower in calories. If you don't want to use a plant stanol margarine, flavor your veggies with fresh lemon, or top them with salsa or one teaspoon of Parmesan cheese. Trust me, if my husband can make the switch, so can you.

Small Change Toppings and Spreads Tips

1. Prepare dips, dressings, and other spreads with low-fat ingredients.

2. Stick to recommended serving sizes—usually, two tablespoons.

3. Swap butter for a margarine that contains plant stanols.

4. Add flavor with herbs, spices, and low-fat condiments (mustards, flavored vinegars, hot sauce, horseradish, salsa).

5. Try hummus on, or in, just about anything.

THE ULTIMATE LOW-FAT TOPPING: HUMMUS

When you're trying to lower your fat intake, hummus is your friend. Made from chickpeas, this Middle Eastern dip/spread can also be used as a condiment in place of fattier toppings like mayonnaise and sour cream. It's tasty, takes only minutes to make, and is virtually fat-free.

Hummus is versatile, too. Experiment with different types of beans (I like black-bean hummus), add fresh veggies (the following recipe contains fresh red bell pepper), and change the seasonings to your taste. Hummus is also delicious on whole-grain crackers. Watch your serving size—two tablespoons will give a burger, sandwich, or even baked potato all the flavor you need! And if you are not the make-at-home type, no worries. So many varieties are available in your local supermarket.

Homestyle Hummus

1 (15-ounce) can garbanzo beans (low-sodium), drained with 1 to 2 tablespoons liquid reserved

1 medium red bell pepper, cut into ½ inch pieces

½ teaspoon ground cumin

2 tablespoons lemon juice

3 cloves garlic, minced

2 tablespoons chopped fresh parsley

Combine all ingredients in a blender or food processor. Blend, adding reserved liquid until the mixture is smooth and creamy. Makes about 2 cups. Store in small container in refrigerator (will last one week) or freezer (2 months).

DISCOVER A NEW "TOPPING": VEGETABLES

A good piece of cheese is one of life's great pleasures and meant to be enjoyed for its own sake. However, somewhere along the line, cheese became an accessory to food—particularly fast food and restaurant-chain food—rather than the star attraction. The result: liquid cheese ladled over French fries, melted over towers of nachos, and draped over ginormous hamburgers.

This small change is simple: Wherever you would add cheese—or other "extras" like bacon on a hamburger, or bacon bits and croutons on a salad—add vegetables instead.

If you eat a salad for your lunch, it's fine to add cheese as your protein. But if you top your salad with grilled chicken also, the cheese is an "extra" because you don't need it for protein. Save it for later and enjoy it as a snack (one ounce) with a serving of whole-grain crackers.

Rather than add or order cheese (or extra cheese) or bacon on a burger, top it with lettuce, tomato, and onion. Again, hummus is another tasty low-fat burger topping, adding extra flavor for a fraction of the fat and calories.

Make sure your veggie toppings are low in fat and calories, however. You defeat the purpose if you smother a steak with butter-sautéed onions and mushrooms, or top your sandwich with too much guacamole or sliced avocado (which is technically a fruit, but you get my meaning).

Veggies are a great topping for pasta, too. Sautéed in a teaspoon of olive oil, with garlic, they add fiber, crunch, and flavor. Can't quite picture it? Experiment! Sauté your favorite veggies—orange or red bell peppers, carrots, broccoli, cauliflower, mushrooms, eggplant, zucchini, green beans, snow peas—in a teaspoon of olive oil. Or grill them. Either result is delicious.

If you like, before you sauté the veggies, sauté onions or minced fresh garlic or ginger to pump up their flavor. As they cook, add basil, parsley, cayenne pepper or red pepper flakes, and oregano or thyme. And yes, when you've piled them on top of your steaming plate of whole-wheat pasta, add a teaspoon of Parmesan for flavor—delicious, filling, and healthy.

While most of my patients increased their vegetable intake without complaint, a few balked at substituting veggies for high-fat toppings ("Don't I eat enough vegetables already?"). Well, not if you want to lose weight. Here are two of the most common rationalizations I've heard:

A salad just isn't a salad without cheese, bacon bits, and croutons.

Small Change Solution: On occasion, a small amount of cheese is fine. I admit to enjoying a bit of feta on my dinner salad once in a while, too! But I use just enough to add flavor. If you use it, use it sparingly—half an ounce, tops. Bacon bits and croutons, however, add a significant amount of fat and calories. So more often than not, cover your salad plate with vegetables, have your dressing on the side, and pass on the high-fat bacon bits and croutons. Once you give them up, you'll see that veggies offer plenty of satisfying crunch and flavor.

I like turkey burgers, but they're so dry. I can't eat them without topping them with a slice or two of cheese.

Small Change Solution: It's true that ground turkey is leaner than ground beef, which makes it a bit less juicy. But you eat turkey burgers because they're lower in fat. So why would you add that fat back by adding cheese? To get the juiciness you crave, top with a tablespoon of hummus, along with lettuce, tomato, and onion. I swear, you won't miss the cheese at all.

Small Change Top-with-Veggies Tips

1. Top burgers with lettuce, tomato, and onion rather than bacon and cheese.

2. Reduce half the serving of meat on your sandwich and replace with lettuce, cucumbers, tomatoes, and onion.

3. Add lots of veggies instead of fatty meats to your pasta.

4. Top an omelet with veggies, rather than cheese.

5. To recapture the crunch of bacon bits and croutons on a salad, use extracrisp veggies such as carrots, celery, and peppers.

ARE YOU READY TO MOVE ON?

At the end of the day, this Small Change measures your willingness to embrace new flavors, make healthy changes, and trade momentary pleasure for a long-term benefit: a slimmed-down you. As delicious as butter, cheese, and *alfredo* sauce are, their flavor pales to how comfortably zipping up your old pair of skinny jeans makes you feel. Take the Small

Change Success Test below to see if you are ready to move on to the next Small Change.

Small Change Success Test

1. Do you ask for dressing, sauce, and gravy on the side?

2. Have you swapped high-fat salad dressings for low-fat alternatives when you dine out, and do you prepare homemade dressings with low-fat ingredients?

3. Do you order lighter sauces when you eat out and defat homemade sauces?

4. Have you lightened your spreads and toppings, either by buying low-fat brands or making them with low-fat ingredients?

5. Do you top burgers, pasta, and other foods with veggies rather than unhealthy fats?

If you answered yes to only three of the items above, stay with this Small Change as long as you need to while you work on the changes that challenge you. Take your time—you'll get there!

If you answered yes to four questions, congratulations. It's time to tackle another Small Change!

SMALL CHANGE 6

▼▲▼▲▼▲▼▲▼

Skinny Your Meat

If you've ever lost weight on a low-carb diet, raise your hand. Now keep it up if you lost weight *and kept it off.*

I'd bet that hand came down pretty quickly.

Low-carb or "caveman" diet plans aside, if you want to lose weight for good, eating Fred Flintstone–size portions of meat isn't the way to go. Yes, meat is an excellent source of protein. Yes, it's a rich source of important minerals like iron and zinc. But meat, especially beef, can be high in saturated fat, which is linked to obesity, cardiovascular disease, and cancer. There are many studies to support this finding, but the primary message is that sitting down to a steak every night benefits neither your waistline nor your heart. And as healthy as fish and poultry can be, frying it or smothering it in cheeses or high-fat sauces negates its benefits.

Must you become a vegetarian? No. You can be a happy—and healthy—carnivore. What matters is how much meat you eat, how often you eat it, and how it is prepared, and the smallest changes can make a big difference.

Hate chicken breast? Enjoy dark meat—just lose the skin. Love pasta sauce with ground meat? Make it with extra-lean ground beef. The only thing you really need to do is reduce your serving size and let veggies take up the slack. Make meat the understudy, rather than the star, of a meal. For example, stir-fry a small amount of steak with carrots, onions, water chestnuts, and bell peppers, and you get all the flavor with a fraction of the fat.

So if you're a die-hard carnivore, relax. The Small Changes in this chapter will allow you to enjoy meat while still losing weight and protecting your health. You'll still be able to enjoy a juicy steak. You just won't have to loosen your belt after you eat it.

Your Small Change Plan

1. Limit your intake of red meat to two servings per week.

2. Eat fish a minimum of twice a week.

3. Remove the skin from chicken and turkey, whether eating out or dining in.

4. Never fry meat or poultry (or order it fried), and trim visible fat before cooking.

5. Aim for one completely meatless meal per week.

RED MEAT: ENJOY IN MODERATION

My beef with red meat (pardon the pun) isn't so much about weight, but health. There's compelling scientific evidence that meat-heavy diets raise the risk of heart disease and cancer, particularly breast and colorectal cancer. In one study published in 2009, researchers asked more than a half-million men and women over the age of fifty about their diet, and then tracked who died over the next ten years. Those who ate about four ounces of beef, lamb, or veal a day—the amount in a quarter-pound burger—were more than 30 percent more likely to die during that period, mostly from heart disease and cancer.

But don't panic. I'm not saying to give up red meat, just to rethink how often you eat it, which cuts you choose, and how much you put on your plate. Most health experts, me included, recommend two servings of red meat a week. That includes leftovers. Let's say you order a steak on Wednesday, eat half (or less—we'll get to serving size in a moment), and take the rest home in a doggie bag. If you eat another serving for dinner on Thursday night, you've had your two servings for the week. Same thing if you make a roast for dinner, have one serving, and pack a roast-beef sandwich for lunch the next day.

Speaking of servings—they're much smaller than most steakhouses would care to admit. Imagine a slightly inflated iPhone. A serving of red meat should be about that size, or 3.5 ounces. At home, it's simple enough to weigh out that much on a food scale, but when was the last time you saw a 3-ounce steak on a menu? Order your steak, eat half, and, I repeat, take the rest home in a doggie bag. If you know you can't resist eating the whole thing, ask your server to have the chef wrap half and to serve you the other half. And if your entrée is served with butter or a sauce, request that it be served on the side.

The cuts of red meat at the supermarket can vary substantially in fat and saturated fat. The USDA defines *lean beef* as having less than 10 grams of total fat, 4.5 grams or less of saturated fat, and less than 95 milligrams of cholesterol per 3½-ounce serving. If you're shopping for steak, choose lean cuts like round, shoulder, strip, tenderloin, or T-bone (and order those cuts when you dine out, too). If you're in the market for a roast, choose arm or chuck shoulder cuts. When you buy hamburger, spend a bit more and opt for 95 percent lean ground beef.

You can go even leaner than that, though—and if you do, you can eat three servings of red meat a week. Extra-lean cuts include top and bottom round, top sirloin steak, and eye of round and bottom round roast. Per serving, all contain less than 5 grams of total fat, 2 grams of saturated fat, and 95 milligrams of cholesterol.

Whichever red meat you choose, trim any fat you see before you cook it, and then broil or grill to remove even more fat. Spice rubs and low-fat/low-sodium marinades can add so many flavors to meat (especially the less expensive cuts) that you won't even miss the fat.

Some of my patients were raised on red meat and find it hard to imagine not eating it every day. If this applies to you, I'll tell you what I tell them: Although you won't eat meat as often, you and your family *can* continue to enjoy it—just on new terms. And many "meat missteps" are easily remedied.

My husband is a meat-and-potato guy, so I serve more meat than I should because I don't want to cook two different meals.

Small Change Solution: You don't have to. First of all, you can *both* eat lean cuts of beef to help reduce calories and saturated fats. It's good for you and good for him, and he can eat as much as he wants, while you stick to the recommended serving size. You can also broil a steak for him at the same time you broil chicken or fish for yourself. (If you make enough chicken or fish for lunch or dinner the next day, you're actually saving time.) Losing weight, and keeping it off, is a matter of finding these simple solutions. You're setting a good example for your husband. Maybe he will eventually want to join you.

I do a lot of summer entertaining and it's so easy to just throw hamburgers and hot dogs on the grill.

Small Change Solution: Agreed! To slash fat and calories, make your burgers from either ground round or sirloin *and* don't make your patties the size of small Frisbees—three ounces is enough. If you enjoy one or two burgers on the weekends (preferably on whole-grain buns, with lettuce, tomato, and low-calorie condiments), it's not a big deal. As for the hot dogs, well, I would suggest eating those less often. You might also try "tofu dogs." Made from soybeans, these "faux dogs" can be surprisingly tasty.

Small Change Red Meat Tips

1. Enjoy red meat twice a week. If you choose extralean cuts, and stick to the appropriate serving size, you can eat it three times a week.

2. A serving of beef is about 3 ounces—the size of a deck of cards.

3. More often than not, choose loin or round cuts.

4. Try bison—it is much lower in fat than many cuts of beef.

5. Broil or grill rather than panfry.

6. Drain the excess fat from ground beef before you add it to a sauce.

7. Leftovers count toward your two servings per week.

8. If you order a red-meat entrée served with a sauce, request the sauce on the side.

What About "The Other White Meat"?

Depending on the cut, a serving of pork can be as lean as a skinless chicken breast or as high in fat and calories as bacon or spareribs. And even the leanest cut will derail your healthy eating plan if it's panfried or drenched in a heavy sauce. To enjoy pork without sabotaging your waistline, follow these tips.

- For the leanest cut, look for the word *loin*, i.e., tenderloin, loin chops, loin roasts.

- Remove most of the external visible fat on the pork before you cook it.

- Cook pork using a low-fat cooking method, including roasting, grilling, broiling, poaching, or braising.

- Pass up high-fat sauces. Rather, flavor pork with herbs and spices. Coriander, cumin, curry powder, dill, garlic, rosemary, sage, savory, and thyme all go well with pork.

- Watch your portions. Like beef, the recommended serving size is three ounces.

GO FISH, GET LEAN

One of my patients, Michael, thirty-nine, works in finance, and part of his "work" is taking clients to dinner. But those nights of lamb chops and mashed potatoes had taken a toll; on his first visit to my office, he weighed 205 pounds. Since we've started working together, he still takes clients to his favorite steakhouse—and, more often than not, chooses fish over meat—but he's lost 22 pounds in fourteen weeks.

High in protein, low in fat and calories, and rich in heart-protecting omega-3 fatty acids, fish—which includes shellfish—is one of the foods I recommend most often to my clients. It's also delicious. As Michael learned, a perfectly broiled piece of salmon can be as tasty as the best beef filet. From tuna fish to fish tacos, lobster and scallops to sushi, fish is what's for dinner if you like to eat smart and eat well.

As healthful as fish is, if you eat too much, you're still consuming fat and calories you don't need. The recommended serving size for fatty fish (salmon, tuna) is three ounces—four ounces if you opt for a white fish like flounder, sole, or tilapia or for shellfish (scallops, shrimp, lobster), which are lower in calories.

How you cook—or order—fish or shellfish counts, too. At home, grill, bake, broil, or poach fish and add flavor with herbs and spices, salsa, or a squeeze of lemon. Opt for cocktail rather than tartar sauce. When you dine out, pass up fried fish (including popcorn shrimp, battered white fish, or clam strips). Skip entrées that feature cream sauces, like Lobster Newburg. Order fish the same way you would cook it at home. Ask that your entrée be prepared without butter, and that butter or cream sauces be served on the side. If you eat lobster or steamers, pass up the melted butter—a squeeze of lemon really does bring out their flavor.

Health experts recommend that you eat seafood twice a week. That doesn't mean you have to *cook* it twice a week. Have a tuna sandwich for lunch on Monday and broiled scallops or a tilapia fillet for dinner on Thursday, and you've met your quota. Or cook fish once—say, a salmon steak or half pound of grilled shrimp. Eat half for dinner, and save the other half for lunch the next day, perhaps in a salad or over pasta.

While some of my patients love fish, others have a limited taste for it, or are reluctant to eat it. Maybe their excuses sound familiar.

The only fish I like are lobster and shrimp, but I can't eat them because I'm watching my cholesterol.

Small Change Solution: Yes you can. While lob-

ster and shrimp are high in cholesterol, dietary cholesterol doesn't raise blood cholesterol—saturated
fat does. Besides, the American Heart Association
recommends consuming no more than 300 milligrams of cholesterol per day. Three ounces of
lobster or shrimp easily fit within these guidelines. Just don't drench them in butter, which can
raise cholesterol. Give them a squeeze of lemon
instead.

I'm afraid to eat fish. Isn't it full of mercury?

Small Change Solution: Most fish and shellfish
contain traces of mercury, which pose little risk
to most people. Fish that contain higher levels of
mercury, however, may harm an unborn baby or
a young child's developing nervous system. So if
you're a woman of childbearing age, pregnant, or
nursing, you can still eat fish; just follow the federal
recommendations below (they apply to young children, too—just serve smaller portions):

1. Avoid shark, swordfish, king mackerel, or
   tilefish. They contain very high levels of
   mercury.

2. Eat up to twelve ounces a week of fish that
   are lower in mercury, including shrimp,
   canned light tuna, salmon, pollock, and

catfish. Albacore tuna contains more mercury than the canned light variety, so limit yourself to six ounces of that per week.

3. If friends or family give you fresh-caught fish, check advisories about the safety of the fish in your local lakes, rivers, and coastal areas. If no advisories are available, eat up to six ounces per week of fish caught in those waters, but don't eat any other fish that week.

Small Change Fish Tips

1. Enjoy fish at least twice a week.

2. Bake, broil, grill, or steam fish, rather than fry it. You may use a teaspoon of olive oil to prepare it.

3. Keep your serving of fatty fish (tuna, salmon) to 3 ounces. You may have 4 ounces of a white fish (flounder, filet of sole, tilapia).

4. Don't drench shrimp or lobster in butter or cream sauces. Use low-fat alternatives, like fresh lemon, instead.

5. Make extra fish for dinner and eat it for lunch the next day.

6. For a quick meal, use canned fish packed in water, including sardines, salmon, or mackerel.

7. If you eat sushi, stay away from fried tempura sushi.

SKINNY YOUR SUSHI

If you love sushi, here's some good news: You don't have to give it up. It definitely fits into a healthy diet. However, because the calories in sushi can vary depending on the dish and how it's prepared, you do need to order smart. Here's how to have your sushi and eat it, too.

- Start your meal with low-calorie miso soup or a side salad of mixed greens with dressing on the side.

- Swap shrimp tempura or soft-shell crab rolls for California or shrimp/cucumber rolls.

- Order sushi made with brown rice if available—not to save calories, but for the health benefits of whole grains.

- Limit yourself to two rolls (yellowtail/scallion,

tuna/avocado, etc.). Also, order only one roll that contains avocado.

- If you order sushi that contains fish eggs (roe), limit yourself to one roll with roe. While roe contains just 20 calories per tablespoon, most rolls that use roe are the specialty kind, which will typically contain more than one table-spoon of roe. (If you eat six or eight pieces, the calories can definitely add up.)

- Avoid sushi prepared with mayonnaise, such as spicy tuna rolls, or added sauce.

- *Note:* If you're pregnant, don't eat raw fish.

POULTRY: USE THE SKINNY STRATEGY

Low in fat and calories and incredibly versatile, chicken and turkey are the old reliables when you're trying to lose weight and eat healthfully. As long as you remove the fattiest part of the bird—the skin—you can eat it every day. You can even enjoy the dark meat (thighs, legs, and drumsticks) pro-vided it's not fried and you remove the skin. The keys: Stick to recommended serving sizes, prepare poultry using low-fat cooking methods, and skip the creamy sauces.

You can eat up to six ounces of poultry a day,

choosing the lower-fat white meat more often than not. As with red meat, your plate should hold around three ounces of poultry—roughly half a boneless, skinless chicken breast, or one chicken leg with thigh, but without skin. That amount should fit in the palm of your hand (remember that the palm of a petite female is smaller than that of a tall man). Reducing your portion size lowers the amount of fat and cholesterol you consume, especially if you choose the leanest poultry (see the table on pages 168–169).

There are plenty of low-fat ways to prepare poultry at home:

Before you cook it, remove the visible fat, including the skin. Then grill, broil, roast, or bake, rather than fry the poultry, adding flavor with herbs, spices, and low-fat marinades.

For an easy way to add flavor, marinate skinned poultry in balsamic vinegar for 20 minutes. Place the chicken in a pan, sprinkle with dried rosemary, and grill, broil, or bake until cooked through.

Or marinate the skinned poultry in olive oil and Dijon mustard. After 20 minutes, remove it and place in a pan. Top with fresh basil and grill, broil, or bake.

Put a whole bird, or parts, on a rack over a baking pan so the fat drips down into the pan. Stir-frying chicken, with the veggies of your choice and a teaspoon of olive oil, is another option.

If you buy ground poultry for chicken burgers, buy ground breast meat only. Ground poultry often contains the skin, so make sure you ask. If you make barbecued chicken, or home-"fried" chicken, remove the skin first. Avoid making chicken dishes with fat-laden sauces including butter or cream, or fricassee, which uses a lot of oil. Baked or roasted chicken is delicious with a few tablespoons of salsa.

When you're dining out, the same rules apply. Choose baked, grilled, or broiled chicken, removing the skin if necessary, even from barbecued or fried chicken. Stir-fried and sautéed chicken with veggies are other tasty options (request that they use as little oil as possible). Pass up chicken entrées that include heavy cream sauces, or request the sauce on the side.

Although poultry is a staple in my patients' diets, they still offer many reasons for not enjoying it more often.

I would eat more chicken, but it just takes too long to cook when I come home from work. It's easier to pick up a pizza.

Small Change Solution: I encourage my patients

who are too tired to cook to pick up a rotisserie
chicken in the deli department of their supermarket—it's quick and easy, not that expensive, and
your family can enjoy it, too. Quarter it (a quarter
is considered around one serving), remove the skin,
throw a veggie and a small baked potato in the microwave, and *voilà*—dinner is served.

I love duck, but it's so high in fat. That means it's off-limits, right?

Small Change Solution: Well, nothing's off-limits,
but duck is higher in fat and cholesterol than
chicken or turkey—and the culprit is the skin. So if
you really love duck, enjoy it on occasion and please
try to remove the skin.

Chicken versus Turkey: Calorie and Fat Comparison

Chicken (3.5 ounces)			
	Calories	Fat (g)	Saturated fat (g)
Breast with skin	197	8	2
Breast without skin	165	3	1
Wing with skin	290	19	5
Leg with skin	232	13	3
Dark meat with skin	253	15	4
Dark meat without skin	205	9	2.5

Turkey (3.5 ounces)			
	Calories	Fat (g)	Saturated fat (g)
Breast with skin	189	7	2
Breast without skin	135	1	0
Wing with skin	229	12	3
Leg with skin	208	10	3
Dark meat with skin	221	12	3.5
Dark meat without skin	162	4	1.5

LOVE BREADED CHICKEN? TRY MY HEALTHY RECIPE

Yes, you can have "fried" or breaded chicken—if you swap the white flour for oats, and use a low-fat cooking method. I use this healthy breading all the time and my family loves it. My version was handed down from my mother, who paired her oats with wheat germ (which you can use, if desired) and a drop of paprika. While this breading can be used in any chicken dish, my recipe uses thin chicken cutlets. If you use thicker, bone-in dark meat, remove the skin first, follow the breading instructions, and bake instead of fry.

Best Breaded Chicken

   ½ cup oats

   ¼ cup ground flaxseed or wheat germ

   Herbs and spices as desired (I typically add 1
      teaspoon of oregano or ½ teaspoon each of
      sage and thyme)

   2 egg whites

   1 pound poultry (approx. 4 skinless chicken
      cutlets)

   1 tablespoon olive oil

Place the oats in a food processor and process
until they have the consistency of flour; place in a
shallow bowl, mix in ground flaxseed and herbs,
and set aside.

Place the egg whites and a drop of water in a
large bowl; stir. Dip chicken into egg whites, then
the flour mixture. Heat the oil in a large skillet
over medium-high heat. When hot, add "breaded"
chicken and cook for about 10 minutes on each
side, until no longer pink. Remove from the pan,
blot any excess oil with a paper towel, and serve.
Serves four.

Small Change Poultry Tips

1. Remove the skin on chicken or turkey before
   you cook it.

2. Broil, grill, or bake chicken, rather than fry it.

3. Keep your serving to around three ounces.

4. Eat more white meat (breast)—it's lower in fat than dark meat (legs, thighs, and drumsticks).

5. If you can't switch from white meat to dark meat, at least remove the skin.

6. Remove the skin from prepared fried chicken.

7. For lighter, healthier "fried" chicken, bread it with whole-wheat flour (season it if you like) and bake it.

8. When you barbecue chicken, remove the skin before cooking and choose a low-fat sauce (see Small Change 5 for ideas).

✔ How's It Going?

Are you recording your daily exercise in your journal? Do you look for opportunities to add extra steps to your day?

GO MEATLESS ONCE A WEEK

Ever have stir-fried tofu, a veggie burger, or "sausage" made from grains? If not, I suggest you give them a try. Going meatless one day a week (or even more often, if you like) gives you the chance to become a culinary adventurer. Explore new foods and flavors and expand your culinary horizons. Besides, meat alternatives like tofu (and its flavorful cousin, tempeh), "mock meat" made from textured soy protein, and the good old humble bean are delicious substitutes for meat. They also happen to be healthful.

Plant protein is low in fat, high in fiber, and contains zero cholesterol. Soy protein, in particular, is packed with isoflavones, which research suggests can help protect against breast and prostate cancers. Of course, to reap the benefits of going meatless, watch serving sizes and use low-fat cooking methods. (Frying tofu in tons of oil or smothering a veggie burger with full-fat cheese kind of defeats the purpose.)

Beans

I absolutely love beans—they're quick, easy, healthful, and delicious, and there's a variety for every culinary mood. One of my favorite quick dinners is to top a baked potato with ½ cup of black beans, a dollop of low-fat sour cream, and plenty of veggies. I also top my serving of whole-wheat pasta with ½ cup of white beans. Canned beans are fine—in fact, the canning process eliminates some of the sugars that result in bloating and gas. Just be sure to rinse them to remove the salt added during processing.   .

Tofu and Tempeh

While both are made from soybeans, the difference between the two is taste. Tofu has no taste of its own; it takes on the flavor of whatever it is cooked with. Tempeh, made from cooked and slightly fermented soybeans (and sometimes grains and spices), has a mild, slightly nutty flavor.

Both tofu and tempeh have many uses and are high in protein and calcium. Look for both in the produce section of your supermarket and be sure to buy the right type of tofu for the dish you're making (see "Tofu 101" on page 176).

Mock Meats

From fajita-flavored veggie burgers to sausage-style links and patties, today's mock meats do a decent job of mimicking the flavor, texture, and look of hamburgers, hot dogs, sausage, bacon, chicken cutlets, and even cold cuts. I love mock chicken tenders—I bake them and eat them "naked" (without sauce), accompanied by a baked potato. But some of my patients use a light dipping sauce and eat them with baked French fries.

If you've never tried mock meats, these ideas can get you started. However, don't depend on mock meats exclusively. Choose natural soy foods, too, like tofu and edamame.

Small Change Meatless Tips

1. Buy, make, or order veggie burgers instead of regular hamburgers.

2. Try using textured soy protein ("crumbles") in place of ground meats for tacos, or add it to pasta sauce to make a "Bolognese."

3. Add beans or edamame (soybeans in the pod, found in the frozen-veggie section) to pasta sauce instead of ground beef.

4. Treat yourself to a "meaty" portabello mushroom burger rather than a hamburger.

5. Enjoy veggie "bacon" or "sausage" with your breakfast egg whites.

6. Stuff a pita with soy "chicken" strips, spinach leaves, and fresh veggies with spicy mustard.

7. If you're really adventurous, try Quorn. This line of meat-free chicken-style nuggets and patties and meat-free hot dogs and meatballs is made with mycoprotein, an edible fungus similar to truffles, morels, and mushrooms.

8. Grill tofu strips and add instead of grilled chicken to a salad.

Many of my patients balk at going meatless one day a week, at least at first. These are some of the alibis I hear.

I hate the taste of tofu.

Small Change Solution: Really? Because by itself, tofu doesn't really have a taste—rather, it takes on the flavors of what it is cooked with. Try marinating it in one tablespoon of low sodium tamari or soy sauce, one tablespoon water, a one-inch piece of peeled, grated fresh ginger, three cloves of minced garlic, and one tablespoon minced fresh or dried cayenne pepper. Then sauté it with your favorite veggies and serve over a serving of brown rice. Simple, low-calorie, and scrumptious.

I thought eating soy could increase the risk of cancer.

Small Change Solution: Soy foods contain isoflavones, or plant estrogens, some of which have weak estrogen activity and—in animal studies—appear to protect against hormone-dependent cancers. However, it's possible that high doses of soy could raise the risk of estrogen-fueled cancers, such as breast or endometrial cancer. If you have breast cancer, consume only moderate amounts of soy foods as part of a healthy, plant-based diet and stick primarily with whole-soy foods such as tofu, soy milk, and edamame rather than processed foods made with soy isolate or isolated soy protein. Avoid soy supplements, which contain high, and possibly dangerous, amounts of isoflavones.

TOFU 101

The first time you shop for tofu, you'll notice that there are quite a few types to choose from: soft, firm, precooked, marinated, even presweetened (for desserts). This cheat sheet will help you choose—and use—different kinds of tofu.

Lesson 1: Tofu comes in two main types. *Regular* tofu is dense and solid and holds up well in stir-fry dishes, soups, or on the grill. Made by a slightly different process, *silken* tofu is creamy—almost like custard—so it's perfect for salad dressings, sauces, even desserts. Both regular and silken tofu are available in soft, medium, firm, and extrafirm consistencies.

Lesson 2: While regular and silken tofu are made from the same ingredients, they are processed differently, so when you're cooking, you cannot exchange one type for another. In other words, don't try to grill silken tofu or make a dip with firm tofu.

Lesson 3: Press and drain tofu before using. This allows it to absorb more flavor when you cook it. Simply place the block of tofu on a cutting board that has been covered with paper towels, cover the tofu with another paper towel, weigh down the block with a heavy bowl, and let the tofu drain for 15 minutes.

If you've never cooked with tofu, you'll be surprised at how versatile it is, and how tasty it can be. These tips can get you started, but you're sure to branch out from here.

- Use tofu instead of chicken in a stir-fry with lots of veggies.

- Add chunks of firm tofu to soups and stews.

- Try marinating tempeh or firm tofu in low-fat barbecue sauce and then grilling it, or cut it into chunks, sauté it, and add it to chili or spaghetti sauce.

- Use tofu to make lasagna and meatballs instead of regular meat.

- Make "egg salad" with tofu chunks, diced celery, low-fat mayonnaise, and spicy brown mustard.

- Substitute puréed silken tofu for all or part of the mayonnaise, sour cream, cream cheese, or ricotta cheese in dips and creamy salad dressings.

ARE YOU READY TO MOVE ON?

If you're a die-hard meat lover, you may have found this Small Change a challenge at first. (Around three ounces of meat? Is she kidding?) But hopefully you've discovered that you can have your beef (or pork, or chicken . . .) and eat it, too, as long as you follow a few simple guidelines. You may even be surprised at just how flavorful skinnying your meat can be! Take the Small Change Success Test below to see if you are ready to move on to the next Small Change.

Small Change Success Test

1. Have you limited your intake of red meat to two servings per week?

2. Do you eat fish at least twice a week?

3. Do you remove the skin from chicken and turkey, whether you're eating at home or at a restaurant?

4. Have you stopped frying meat, fish, or poultry (or ordering it fried), and do you trim visible fat before cooking?

5. Are you trying to go completely meatless one day per week?

If you answered yes to only three of the items on this chapter's Small Change Success Test, stay with this Small Change as long as you need to while you work on the changes that challenge you. Take your time—you'll get there!

If you answered yes to four questions, congratulations. It's time to tackle another Small Change!

▼▲▼▲▼▲▼▲▼▲▼

Eat the Right Kinds (and Amounts) of Fat

When I counsel patients, I always make sure they understand that eating fat doesn't make you fat. The culprit is eating *too much* or too little fat.

Yes, it's true: If you don't eat enough fat—or any fat, for that matter—you're in danger of gaining weight. If you're thinking *Huh?*, let me explain. Dietary fat promotes satiety—that full, satisfied feeling that lets you know you've had enough to eat. If you eat a meal especially low in fat, or worse, contains no fat at all, don't be surprised if, in a few hours, you find your hand in the cookie jar. Without fat in your diet, you're more likely to be constantly hungry and to overeat.

The lesson here? You can follow an ultra low-fat diet and still end up hungry, miserable . . . and fatter. I thought Americans had learned this lesson after the low-fat craze of the 1990s, but unhappily, not everyone got the memo. We forgot about calories and just counted fat grams. So we would chow down on a whole sleeve of fat-free cookies, forgetting that while they may have been fat-free, they still contained sugar . . . otherwise known as calories. Also, when people avoid fat, most reach for carbs because they feel they are lower in fat (pretzels rather than chips, for example). But then they'll eat too many, because there's no fat to provide satiety and fill them up.

When I work with "fat phobics," I tell them that adding a tablespoon of peanut butter or a slice of avocado to their diet may actually help them lose weight. One of my patients, Allison, twenty-eight, is a former fat phobic. "The word alone frightened me," she said. "Just thinking about it, I felt myself packing on the pounds." But I convinced her to incorporate fats into her diet, insisting that she could return to her fruits and vegetables if the extra pounds started creeping on.

Once she began including healthy fats like avocado, nuts, and feta cheese into her diet, Allison reconsidered her fear. "Not only did I not gain weight . . . I *lost* weight! Needless to say, fats are no longer my enemy but an essential part of my diet."

QUALITY COUNTS AS MUCH AS QUANTITY

Fats are an essential part of everyone's diet. Fats are a rich source of energy (nine calories per gram) and essential fatty acids, which your body needs for optimal health and well-being. *Essential* means that the body cannot produce them itself and has to take them in from the food you eat. And let's face it—most foods taste better with a little fat. For example, a salad dressed with olive oil and balsamic vinegar is far more satisfying than a salad dressed with the vinegar alone. Finally, fat-soluble vitamins such as D, K, E, and A are absorbed more efficiently in the body if they're eaten with a little fat. Eating a salad dressing that contains a healthy fat is a win-win situation.

All that being said, not all fats are equally healthy. A porterhouse steak, avocado, salmon, and doughnuts all contain a large amount of dietary fat. But the steak and doughnuts contain *saturated* fats, known to drive up total cholesterol levels, clog arteries, and promote heart disease and some cancers. By contrast, the *unsaturated* fats in the avocado and salmon may actually do your body good, helping to prevent and treat heart disease, diabetes, cancer, and obesity.

Specifically, avocado is rich in an unsaturated fat called *monounsaturated fat*, also found in nuts and seeds and olive and canola oils. Salmon is an excellent source of *omega-3 fatty acids*, another healthy fat found primarily in fatty, cold-water fish as well as in flaxseeds and their oil.

The not-so-healthy fats include saturated and trans fats. Animal foods—pork chops, dark meat poultry with skin, whole milk and full-fat cheese, bacon, and butter—are high in saturated fats, as are the coconut and palm oils often used in processed foods. Trans fats are found in store-bought baked goods, a lot of fried foods such as doughnuts and French fries, and some margarines.

Here's the good news: Opt for the healthier fats (and enjoy them in moderation), and you'll feel satisfied after every meal and snack. You won't overeat. You'll benefit your health. And yes, you'll even lose weight.

Your Small Change Plan

1. Limit your fat intake to 25 percent of your daily calories.

2. Upgrade your oils.

3. Limit full-fat cheese to one serving a day.

4. Terminate trans fats.

FAT: NOT TOO LITTLE—OR TOO MUCH

As mentioned, some people are afraid to consume any fat at all. Others think they can eat as much "healthy fat" as they want. And too many unknowingly consume far too much. What do they have in common? All of them have a tough time eating healthfully and losing weight.

Knowing how much fat to eat—and which kinds to choose most often—isn't rocket science. I've spent most of the book discussing small choices that add up to big weight loss. Most of the Small Changes add up to this: Opt for lean, lower-fat, and fat-free alternatives to high-fat and -calorie fare, and you won't have to spend much time thinking about fat grams.

That said, as a general guideline, consume about 25 to 30 percent of your daily calories from fat, and make sure the majority are the healthy unsaturated fats (monounsaturated, polyunsaturated, and omega-3 fats, rather than saturated fats). If you eat about 1,600 calories a day, that means 400 calories, or about 44 grams of fat (1 gram of fat contains 9 calories), and only 7 percent of those 400 calories should come from saturated fat.

Keep in mind, however, that losing weight and keeping it off isn't about counting fat grams (or carbs, or calories, for that matter) each day. It's about creating that healthy plate. When it comes to fat, picture your healthy plate, then picture a napkin ring beside it. That's your mini "plate" for fat.

With fat, as with every other food, portion size matters, and it's important to be aware of how much fat you use. Every meal can be prepared with some fat, but if you sauté veggies in olive oil, add cheese to your dinner salad, and then eat a food that contains fat naturally, like a piece of salmon or a sirloin steak, you're eating too much fat, whether it's healthy fat or not. Basically, you want to eat one serving of fat with a meal, not three. So when it comes to fat, you need to eat less fat in general, choose the healthy ones in particular, and steer clear of the fatty pitfalls below.

I really love avocado, especially in guacamole, but avocados contain so much fat. I never eat either of them.

Small Change Solution: Good news—you can enjoy them again! Avocado and guacamole are not the enemy, nor is any monounsaturated fat. The key is serving size. If you're like most of my patients, you think one serving of avocado is the entire avocado, but in reality, it's one-fifth of the fruit; and one serving of guacamole is two tablespoons. The best part is, when you eat them, you're not eating other unhealthier fats, like butter or trans fats. So enjoy avocados in moderation.

I know nuts are healthy, and include lots of them in my diet every day. But I still can't seem to lose weight. Maybe I should give them up?

Small Change Solution: There's no reason to eliminate nuts from your diet, but you may be over-doing it, which is slowing up your weight loss. Just because a food is good for you doesn't mean that eating more of it will make you healthier. Some-times it just makes you heavier! One thing I always tell my patients: Never eat nuts from the jar or container. It's too easy to overeat. Measure out one serving (one ounce = visually a shot glass full) first, then enjoy!

The Small Change tips below should go a long way toward helping you stay within your 25 percent goal. As always, unless you're eating veggies pre-pared without fat, *watch your portion sizes*!

Small Change "Just Right" Fat Tips

1. Identify the food that naturally contains fat in your meal prior to cooking, and stick to the serving size (i.e., 3 ounces of salmon).

2. Choose just one serving of added fat per meal (i.e., avocado on your turkey sandwich, cheese in your egg white omelet, veggies sautéed in olive oil).

3. If you like a variety of added fat with your meals, use less than the actual serving sizes. For example, use 1 teaspoon of oil on your fish and 1 teaspoon on your veggie (versus 1 tablespoon on each), and add ½ ounce of cheese to your salad rather than 1 ounce.

4. When dining out, request that salad dressings, sauces, and gravies be served on the side, then use only part of the portion you're given, since it's nearly guaranteed they are giving you more than one serving of fat.

5. Measure out a serving of nuts or seeds before you eat them.

OPT FOR THE HEALTHIEST OILS

Often, when I work with patients, I'm happy to see that their food journals contain a lot of veggies and salads. I'm also happy to see that they're choosing unsaturated oils, like olive, canola, and flaxseed. I feel like they've heard my main message: Healthful food doesn't have to be tasteless.

As I said at the start of this change, even a little fat adds big flavor and delight to a meal or a dish. For years, I dressed my salads only with balsamic vinegar—no oil. I enjoyed the taste, or thought I did. Gradually, however, when I went out to dinner, I began to order salad dressing on the side—some absolutely delicious dressings. My balsamic-only dressing began to bore me. I still love balsamic vinegar, but for me it really is better paired with olive oil.

Some of my patients, however, love oil too much. Lots of times they aren't aware of how much they're using. So when they come for their follow-up appointments and aren't losing weight, I tend to find that they are not only using oil on their dinner salad but also smothering their veggies or broiled fish or chicken with it.

The moral of the story: When it comes to healthy fats—and oil is most definitely a fat—while quality counts, quantity counts, too. And unless you measure it out, you might be consuming a lot more oil—and calories—than you think. But do use some. If you don't, there's a good chance you'll still be hungry after your meal, and overeat later on.

Once you get a handle on how much oil to use, you'll want to match the right oil to the right foods and cooking techniques. Be adventurous and try oils you've never tasted. If you're used to plain old corn oil, I think you'll be pleasantly surprised! Here's a cheat sheet:

For salads, olive, sunflower, safflower, flaxseed, or walnut oils are excellent choices. With the exception of extra-virgin olive oil, olive oil has a robust flavor, while sunflower oil (pressed from the seeds) and safflower oil (pressed from a thistle-type flower) have a delicate taste and a lighter texture. If you opt for sunflower oil, you can get either high-oleic sunflower oil, which has monounsaturated levels of 80 percent and above, or the more common linoleic sunflower oil, which is high in polyunsaturates or linoleic acid, an essential fatty acid.

Flaxseed's rich, nutty taste adds a pleasant flavor to a salad, and it's a rich source of alpha-linolenic acid (ALA), which your body converts into omega-3s. It goes rancid quickly—high or even room temperatures destroy its fragile structure—so keep it in the refrigerator and use it within a few months of opening. Walnut oil is best used uncooked or in cold sauces because it becomes slightly bitter when heated.

For stir-frying, stick with sesame and peanut oils.

Both can be heated to high temperatures without smoking or breaking down. Made from roasted sesame seeds, sesame oil has a strong, smoky flavor, while peanut oil has a light, nutty taste. Opt for peanut oil if you're using strong ingredients such as ginger or chili paste.

For sautéing veggies, olive, canola, and soybean oils win high marks. When it comes to olive oil, extra-virgin is the highest quality—it tends to be higher in polyphenols (a powerful antioxidant) than refined brands. You might buy a less expensive (but often less flavorful) virgin olive oil for cooking and invest in the pricier and more flavorful virgin or extra-virgin oils for using in vinaigrettes or drizzling over steamed veggies. If you prefer less strongly flavored oil, opt for soybean or canola.

Whether they fear using oil or use too much, my patients have their stories to tell:

Even though it's high in saturated fat, I use coconut oil because I heard it can promote weight loss.

Small Change Solution: Yes, a few books have touted coconut oil as a way to help you lose weight. Their authors claim that coconut oil can provide a feeling of fullness and reduce cravings for carbs and sweets. The reason? Because—and this is only a theory—coconut oil is made up of medium-chain fatty acids, which are shorter than the long-chain fatty acids in veggie oils and meat. So although coconut oil is technically a saturated fat, the body breaks it down faster than it breaks down a pork chop. Yet because it is high in fat, coconut oil makes you feel full, so you eat less. Researchers at McGill University in Canada conducted a study in 2002 that seems to support this claim.

However, when it comes to weight loss, there are no miracles, and regardless of its fatty acid makeup, coconut oil is still packed with saturated fat—92 percent saturated fat, in fact, even more than in butter (66 percent saturated fat). In moderation, no problem. But in large amounts, saturated fats can lead to high cholesterol and heart disease. Bottom line: You like coconut oil, have a little coconut oil. But don't think having a lot of coconut oil is going to be a health cure or a weight-loss miracle, because it doesn't work that way. You have to eat healthfully, practice portion control, and get active.

I'd use olive oil, but it's too expensive!

Small Change Solution: Olive oil *is* typically pricier than corn oil or plain old vegetable oil. However, since you'll be using it by the teaspoon, you can get a smaller bottle, which should last you a while.

But if you're on a budget, there are other healthful oils besides extra-virgin olive oil. In fact, the only reason to buy olive oil is if you enjoy the taste. If you don't, canola oil is just as healthy and has a more neutral flavor. You can also get olive oil blends—extra-virgin olive oil mixed with the more inexpensive canola oil—or simply buy canola oil.

Small Change Healthy-Oils Tips

1. Keep in mind that one serving of olive oil is a tablespoon.

2. Fill a mister (available at most kitchen stores) with your favorite cooking oil and mist rather than pour oil on veggies, pasta, and fish. Or use cooking oil sprays. You are guaranteed to use less.

3. Whether you broil, grill, or sauté fish, poultry, or veggies, use heart-healthy oils instead of butter.

4. If you need to eyeball the recommended amount of oil, 1 teaspoon is about the size of one playing dice. Limit yourself to 3 teaspoons per day.

5. When dining out, request that a side dish or entrée be prepared with a small amount of olive oil instead of butter.

DON'T FORGET THESE HEALTHY FATS

There's a reason that health experts recommend eating omega-3–rich fish twice a week. Our bodies need essential fatty acids to function normally. Essential fatty acids EPA (eicosapentaenoic acid) and DHA (docosahexaenoic acid) are not made in the body. So to get them, we need to eat them in food or take them as supplements.

Research has linked EPA and DHA with heart health, including lowering blood pressure and triglyceride levels, stabilizing life-threatening irregular heart rhythms, and preventing the gunk in arteries (plaque) from breaking away from the lining of arteries and causing a heart attack or stroke. Other studies show that omega-3s may help with a variety of conditions, including rheumatoid arthritis and depression.

The best way to get these healthy fats is to eat fish. Anchovies, bluefish, herring, mackerel, salmon, sardines, sturgeon, lake trout, and tuna are particularly high in EPA and DHA. Plant foods also contain omega-3s. Walnuts, flax and flaxseed oil, canola oil, olive oil, and soybeans are good sources of ALA, which the body converts into DHA and EPA. However, plant sources of omega-3s may not offer the same benefits as those found in fish.

To raise your intake of omega-3s simply and safely, follow the guidelines on the next page.

- Eat fish at least twice a week, particularly those rich in EPA and DHA.

- If you absolutely won't touch fish, eat flax-seed—rich in ALA, it's the most potent plant form of omega-3s there is. Other sources of omega-3s include canola oil, walnuts, broccoli, cantaloupe, kidney beans, and cauliflower.

- If possible, opt for grass-fed poultry and beef. They have much higher levels of omega-3s than animals that are fed conventional grains.

- Some fatty fish, including wild swordfish, tilefish, and shark, contain high levels of toxins, including mercury and PCBs. Don't eat more than seven ounces of these fish a week, and children and pregnant women shouldn't eat them at all.

- Before you take an omega-3 supplement, talk to your doctor. Depending on your health or any medications you take, it may not be right for you.

✔ **How's It Going?**

Are you noting the time that you eat your meals and snacks in your food journal? Has it helped you not to go too long without eating between meals?

GO EASY ON THE CHEESE

For foodies, there's virtually nothing better on earth than the flavor and texture of a good full-fat cheese. But there can be too much of a good thing. Average U.S. cheese consumption nearly tripled between 1970 and 2003, from 11 pounds per person to 31 pounds. In 1980, Americans ate 17.5 pounds of cheese per person per year. By 2007, we were eating just shy of 33 pounds of the stuff!

That's a lot of cheese—and a lot of calories. What's more, the full-fat variety is packed with saturated fat, which raises heart-disease risk. The good news is, you don't have to give it up; just eat it in moderation. (And while you'll want to limit full-fat cheese, there's no need to limit low-fat dairy—you can still enjoy low-fat yogurt, cottage cheese, or milk.)

For those times when you just must have real cheese, have it—an ounce, once a day. Splurge on really good cheese, because when it comes to flavor, a little goes a long way, so an ounce is enough.

I tell my patients to opt for a hard cheese with strong flavor (for instance, Parmesan, Romano, or feta), and grate it into pasta, salad, and soup. My personal favorite is feta. I love it on salad, in a veggie omelet, on pizza instead of mozzarella, and with white beans and spinach on whole-wheat pasta. Sometimes I actually use less than an ounce because it's so flavorful, and many of my "cheeseaholic" patients use feta on their salads now as well. Another way to practice portion control is to buy presliced cheese (have one slice), string cheese, cheese cubes, or individually wrapped single-serving cheese, rather than whole blocks of cheese. That way, you don't cut off—and eat—more than an ounce, and when you eat one piece of string cheese, or count out how many cubes equal one serving (four), you know you're not overdoing it.

Once you've enjoyed your ounce a day, you can opt for healthy alternatives to full-fat cheese. There are plenty of them, all delicious. I've discussed them throughout the book, but you'll find some of them again in the upcoming Small Change tips. However, you might be filled with some misgivings, just like my patients:

I hate the taste of fat-free cheese, so I'd rather not eat cheese at all.

Small Change Solution: Whoa—who said you had to eat fat-free cheese? Forget about it, especially if you don't like it. But low-fat cheese is another story. For one thing, a little bit of fat helps fill you up. For another, if you haven't tried low-fat cheese lately, the flavor has vastly improved over the years. You may need to try a few brands before you settle on one you like. If you don't find one you like, don't sweat it. Enjoy your ounce of full-fat cheese a day.

I got into the habit of eating a lot of cheese when I was on a low-carb diet—it was the only thing that really filled me up. I don't think I can limit myself to only an ounce of cheese a day!

Small Change Solution: Full-fat cheese helps fill you up because of its protein and fat content—but along with that full tummy, you're getting way too much saturated fat and calories, especially if you're slicing cheese off a block, rather than stopping at one serving.

Low-fat cheese, and other low-fat dairy, can satisfy you, too. Rather than reach for whole-fat cheese when your stomach rumbles, add a serving of low-fat yogurt or cottage cheese to your meals instead. I'm betting that you'll feel just as satisfied.

Small Change Ease-Up-on-Cheese Tips

1. Limit yourself to 1 ounce of full-fat cheese a day. After that, try other low-fat dairy options, like yogurt or cottage cheese.

2. Instead of adding 2 or 3 slices of cheese to a sandwich, add a serving of avocado instead.

3. Rather than add shredded cheese to a salad, add flavor and crunch with an ounce of chopped almonds, pecans, or walnuts.

4. Stuff your omelet with veggies—onions, peppers, spinach, mushrooms—instead of cheese.

5. If you tend to get hungry at night, have your cheese serving for your midafternoon snack with a piece of fruit or a serving of whole-grain crackers, to hold you over until dinner.

AVOID THE TRANS FAT TRAP

When I was the host of *Diet Diva*, we did an episode about making breakfast for dinner, so I made a delicious egg white omelet with veggies and whole-wheat toast. I also recommended a certain brand of tofu cream cheese. Because it contained less saturated fat than butter, I told viewers that it was a healthier substitution—the less saturated fat you eat, the better. The next day, a viewer e-mailed me. She'd intended to buy the tofu cream cheese, she wrote, but it contained trans fats. I was shocked—

I had the same brand in my refrigerator at home! Sure enough, when I checked the Nutrition Facts label, one serving of my "healthy choice" contained two grams of trans fat!

This story illustrates how important it is to read a food's ingredients label to avoid these unhealthy fats, which are as bad for your health as they are for your waistline.

Trans fats are created by adding hydrogen to liquid vegetable oils, which makes them more solid. Companies like trans fats because they give foods a pleasant taste and texture, and restaurants and fast-food outlets like oils with trans fats because they can be used over and over again in commercial fryers. (Yuck.)

Trans fats deliver a double whammy: unlike other fats, trans fats both raise your "bad" (LDL) cholesterol and lower your "good" (HDL) cholesterol. A diet high in trans fats raises your risk of heart disease, stroke, and type 2 diabetes. While some meat and dairy products, including beef, lamb, and butterfat, naturally contain small amounts of trans fats, it isn't known whether they have the same bad effects on cholesterol as those that are manufactured.

There are a few good ways to escape the trans fat trap. The fail-safe way is to stick with whole, natural foods, as I've been suggesting all along. The

fewer ingredients a food lists on its label, the better!
Another way is to limit your consumption of packaged cookies, cakes, doughnuts, and other sweets as
well as salty packaged snack foods. And because so
many fast-food restaurants are still using hydrogenated oils in their fryers, the less often you go and
the more meals you prepare at home, the better.
These strategies will not only protect your heart but
also definitely benefit your waistline.

As my own story suggests, however, the best way
to avoid the trap is to read a product's Nutrition
Facts label. Look for the word *hydrogenated* or the
phrase *partially hydrogenated* vegetable oil on the
ingredients label. Another clue: the word *shortening*.
Shortening contains some trans fat. In fact, even if
the Nutrition Facts label says the food contains "0
grams" of trans fat, be wary of how many servings
you eat daily. In the United States, any food can
claim to have no trans fat if it contains under 0.5
grams per serving. While that's a very small amount,
if you eat different foods that all contain less than
0.5 grams of trans fat—or eat multiple servings of
just one food with that small amount, it all adds up.

It's easy to see fat in greasy French fries or a
creamy dressing. Trans fats are not as easy to sleuth
out, as even I discovered. While I always encourage
my patients to opt for whole foods, some still grab

the more convenient processed fare. I definitely understand the need for convenience, as long as they (and you!) understand the need to limit the trans fats.

I've done a lot of reading on how unhealthy trans fats are, so I switched back to butter for my morning toast.

Small Change Solution: I can see your reasoning, but the fact remains that butter is very high in saturated fats. If you really love butter and can't imagine living without it, don't. Just monitor how much you consume. One pat of butter, which is one serving, is equal to the tip of your thumb. If you can spread that on your toast, go for it—many of my patients do. If you can't, spread your toast with a serving of one of the tastiest healthy fats there is: natural peanut butter. It even contains a bonus: protein. I'd bet that you won't even miss the butter.

I know I need an afternoon snack, and for me, it's chips. They're convenient, and I enjoy them. If I only eat them once a day, does it really matter if they contain trans fats?

Small Change Solution: Every once in a while, any food is okay, even one that contains trans fats. But to lose weight and live a longer, healthier life, trans fats need to be eaten less, and healthy fats—and healthy snacks—more. So enjoy your chips (or cookies, or whatever), as long as you eat one serving, and as long as the brand you choose contains no trans fats. Check the Nutrition Facts label for those code words *hydrogenated* or *partially hydrogenated*. If you see them, choose another brand.

However, I suggest trying to give up packaged snack foods in general, because they probably have more calories and less nutrients than most unprocessed choices anyway. Instead, snack on a serving of unsalted nuts or low-fat yogurt and a piece of fruit, or low-fat cheese and whole-grain crackers, checking the label, of course, to make sure the crackers are truly made with whole grains and don't contain trans fats.

Small Changes Trans Fat Tips

1. Read the Nutrition Facts labels on the foods you buy and avoid those that list hydrogenated oils or partially hydrogenated oils.

2. Limit or avoid packaged snack foods and opt for natural snacks that contain healthier fats, such as nuts, seeds, and natural nut butters.

3. Choose a soft tub margarine rather than stick margarine and look for brands with no trans fats.

4. Sauté foods in olive oil instead of margarine.

5. Limit fast-food meals, especially anything fried. More often than not, order a side salad instead of French fries.

ARE YOU READY TO MOVE ON?

Whether you fear eating fat, or fear you can't stop eating it, this Small Change is definitely one of the biggies, for your health as well as your weight. But it's also an interesting one because you'll get to experience new flavors and foods as you knock off extra pounds. The biggest change: eating more whole foods and fewer packaged ones to limit your intake of trans fats. But as with all my Small Changes, this one is a process, not an event, so every small victory counts. Take the Small Change Success Test below to see if you are ready to move on to the next Small Change.

Small Change Success Test

1. Are you limiting your fat intake to 25 percent of your daily calories?

2. Are you using only healthy unsaturated oils, both in cooking and on salads and veggies?

3. Have you limited full-fat cheese to one serving a day?

4. Are you reading ingredients labels carefully, and eliminating foods that contain trans fats as much as possible?

If you answered yes to only one or two of the items in this chapter's Small Change Success Test, keep trying! It's not easy to stick to an ounce of full-fat cheese a day if you're used to eating as much of it as you want, or peering at food labels to sleuth out trans fats. But after a while, you'll get used to it, and you'll be able to take satisfaction in making changes that benefit your health as well as your weight.

If you've answered yes to at least three questions, congratulations. It's time to tackle another Small Change!

▼▲▼▲▼▲▼▲▼

Tame Your Sweet Tooth and Your Saltshaker

Everyone experiences food cravings, and my patients are no exception. Time and again, they describe innocently going about their day, minding their own business, when they're hit by an overpowering desire for chocolate. Or chips. Next thing they know, they're standing in front of the vending machine or are out the door to the nearest deli.

Why are we plagued with cravings? Scientific theories abound—hormones, fluctuations in blood sugar levels, negative emotions like loneliness and anger. But in my view, you don't need to know *why* you have cravings. You need to know how to handle them. You need a plan, and that plan comes down to two words: *be prepared*.

Often, cravings stem from a purely physical reason: hunger. Maybe it's been more than four hours since your last meal. For example, mid-afternoon cravings, which are quite common, are the body's way of saying, "Hey, it's been a while since lunch." Hunger might turn to craving if you didn't eat enough at a certain meal, or that meal didn't contain enough fat and protein, which promote a feeling of fullness that lasts longer than a meal composed primarily of carbohydrates.

Most of the time, however, cravings begin in your head. Emotions can play a big part in cravings. Negative feelings like stress, boredom, or loneliness can trigger them. So can childhood memories of how good certain foods made us feel—the chocolate cake Mom used to bake, the pasta dished up by your grandmother. Sensory triggers, such as smells and visual cues, can also set off cravings. As you pass the cinnamon-bun stand or pizza place in the mall, chances are your mouth will water. Or we crave foods we "shouldn't" eat—those dark, evil, "forbidden" foods like doughnuts, chocolate, or pizza. (Yes, I'm kidding.)

One thing we do know about cravings: They tend to hit less when you eat regular balanced meals, including breakfast and healthy snacks. (Now may be a good time to revisit Small Change 1's healthy eating schedule.) Exercise may also help control cravings. Research has shown that regular exercise releases feel-good brain chemicals called endorphins into the body, which boost your mood and reduce stress.

It's okay to give in to your cravings once in a while, as long as you make a *conscious decision* to indulge them, rather than get blindsided by them. If you accept cravings as a normal part of life, and have a plan to deal with them, they won't sabotage your eating plan or derail your weight loss. The Small Changes in this chapter will help you deal with cravings, so they don't deal with you. But to use them, you first need to identify exactly what it is that you crave.

SWEET OR SALTY? CREAMY OR CRUNCHY?

You may love jelly doughnuts. You may, at times, even crave them. But if you try to satisfy a craving for pizza with a jelly doughnut, there's a good chance you'll continue to eat until you succumb to the doughnut—or a healthy alternative.

To avoid a scenario like that, it's critical to identify *exactly* what it is that you want. This helps you form a rational response. Do you want sweet or salty? Do you crave a specific food, like chocolate-covered pretzels, or just a general "something sweet"?

Once you've identified whether you want sugar or salt, drill down a bit more. Do you want a creamy texture or a crunchy one? Low-fat chocolate pudding or ice cream can satisfy a sweet and creamy, while a granola bar may soothe a sweet-and-crunchy craving. Hummus or a creamy soup made with low-fat ingredients might satisfy a yen for a salty yet creamy food, while baked chips or pretzels could satisfy a taste for both crunch and salt. If you take thirty seconds to ponder these two categories—sweet or salt, creamy or crunchy—you probably won't nibble endlessly on a little of this, a little of that, which can add up to *a lot* of calories.

Once you know what you crave, you have a decision to make. Will you eat it, or make a healthy substitution?

If you decide to indulge your craving, go for it. Just stick to the recommended serving size. For example, if you crave ice cream, have ½ cup, not the whole half gallon. Enjoy one slice of pizza, not four. Splurge on a small serving of fast-food fries, not the extralarge. You'll be surprised at how satisfying that one serving can be.

Sometimes, you don't even need to eat the whole thing. My husband and I have a favorite restaurant that serves a fabulous chocolate layer cake. While

I'm not a chocolate fanatic, going to this restaurant actually triggers a craving for this specific cake. So every time we dine there, which is often, we order a slice for dessert. The slices are huge—enough for six people, no exaggeration. I savor four forkfuls and, just like that, my craving is satisfied. My husband eats his share, and then we ask the waiter to take away the rest.

If you know one serving won't quench your craving, identify a low-fat, low-calorie alternative that will satisfy you. For example, if a small square of chocolate won't make a dent in your lust for chocolate, maybe a sugar-free hot chocolate, low-fat chocolate milk or pudding, or a low-fat frozen fudge bar will. It sounds counterintuitive to say that a healthy alternative will cool your desire for an unhealthy one. If the food you crave triggers overeating, avoid it, or make do with a substitute.

Your Small Change Plan

1. HALT cravings in their tracks.

2. Prepare yourself for midday cravings: Eat an adequate, satisfying breakfast and lunch and arm yourself with healthy snacks.

3. To short-circuit nighttime cravings, eat an adequate, satisfying dinner, consider eating your evening meal later, and plan for a healthy snack.

4. If you overindulge, get back on track.

HALT CRAVINGS IN THEIR TRACKS

When you're in a weakened state, either physically or emotionally, it's harder to resist temptation. The solution: Don't let yourself get in a weakened state.

HALT, an acronym for Hungry, Angry, Lonely, and Tired, is a popular slogan in recovery communities like Alcoholics Anonymous and Overeaters Anonymous. The idea is that each of these four conditions, if not taken care of, can lead to relapse. But this powerful technique also works to short-circuit food cravings. It's simple to use. Just ask yourself the questions below.

"Am I physically hungry?" True hunger is natural. It comes on gradually, grows more intense the longer you go without food, and goes away when you eat. If you *are* hungry, eat a healthy snack to tide you over until your next meal. If you're *not* hungry, continue

with the questions—they'll help you find a calorie-free way to meet your emotional need.

"Am I angry?" Eating an entire sleeve of Oreos because you're mad at your mother, your partner, or your boss may mask your anger, but it won't get rid of it. Besides, you know you'll feel guilty and furious with yourself later on. Why put yourself through that? Choose a healthy way to blow off steam; take a brisk walk if possible or let it all out in your journal.

"Am I lonely?" No matter how delicious it is, food is no substitute for human companionship. To get the true connection you seek, call a friend or relative, or better yet, make plans to get together for a (healthy) dinner, a movie, or to simply hang out.

"Am I tired?" You can't make smart choices about food if you're nodding off. Catch a twenty-minute catnap, take a quick shower, or—if it's nighttime—head to bed. Yes, it really is that simple. You can't eat if you're sleeping!

I encourage my patients to pinpoint the emotion that lies beyond their "craving." Simply knowing you're not hungry, but rather bored, lonely, stressed, or frustrated can extinguish the craving.

You might also find it helpful to keep a food/mood journal. Each time you experience a craving, write down the time it occurred, the main emotion associated with it, the food you craved, and what you did about it (resisted or gave in). In time, you may discover a pattern to your cravings, and the feelings that accompany them, that can help you to break the pattern.

My patients often tell me their cravings are beyond their control. Really? They have that little willpower? No way. I tell them that they can take back their power simply by pausing, trying to figure out what they're feeling, and consciously deciding whether to resist or give in.

I can't kick my cravings no matter how hard I try. I think I'm addicted to sugar.

Small Change Solution: Some researchers are exploring the possibility of sugar addiction. I personally don't subscribe to this theory, but if it were true, you'd need to eliminate sugar from your diet altogether, as you would cigarettes or alcohol. My take: Maybe if you don't fight your craving for sugar, you'll find that there is a place for it in your diet.

The American Heart Association recommends that the amount of added sugars you consume be no more than half of your daily discretionary calories. For most women, that's about 100 calories per day, or about six teaspoons of sugar. That's the amount in about five chocolate kisses. (For men, it's 150 calories per day, or about nine teaspoons.)

So if you currently resist *all* sugar, consider

giving in to your craving for it—in the recommended amounts. Just make sure the food you crave isn't a "trigger food" (one that leads to overeating), eat a healthy well-balanced diet, and don't swap healthy foods for sugary ones.

I've been under so much stress lately. I deserve a little reward.

Small Change Solution: Food is not a reward. I repeat: *Food is not a reward.* In fact, "rewarding" yourself with food may add to your stress the next time you try to squeeze into your jeans. If you want to reward yourself, schedule a manicure, facial, or massage or take a yoga class. Or simply take a nice long walk.

Small Change HALT Plan

1. Use the HALT technique anytime a craving hits.

2. If you're truly physically hungry, reach for a healthy snack to tide you over until your next meal.

3. If you're not experiencing actual hunger, and can identify what you're feeling as anger, loneliness, or fatigue, take one positive action to meet that need.

DITCH CRAVINGS WITH THE FIVE D'S

Does your mouth water when you pass that dough-nut shop on the way to work? Do you crave a par-ticular food when you go to a particular restaurant, or chips when you watch TV? If so, you may be *conditioned* to respond to certain smells, images, or activities. In other words, you react like a dog.

Remember Pavlov's dogs? In the early 1900s, scien-tist Ivan Pavlov trained dogs to salivate at the sound of a bell. Pavlov knew that dogs naturally salivated when they were fed meat. To condition this response, Pavlov rang a bell each time he fed them. After a while, the dogs salivated when they heard the bell, but *before* they saw the meat. They'd become *conditioned* to expect meat when they heard the tinkle of the bell.

The lesson here: Anything you can do to distract yourself from smells, images, activities, or emotions you associate with your craved foods will help you withstand them. To sever that conditioned response, try the Five D's technique. Use it anytime a craving hits. (The one exception: if it's been more than three hours since your last meal. In that case, reach for a healthy snack to tide you over until your next meal.)

1. **Delay** your urge to cave in to the craving. Drink a tall glass of water. That minute or two can help you reach the next *D*.

2. **Determine** what's going on. Ask yourself, "Why do I want this chocolate chip cookie or this slice of pizza? Am I physically hungry? What else might I really want or need?"

3. **Distract** yourself for 10 minutes. Wait it out. Some experts call this urge-surfing—riding the tumultuous waves of a craving until they subside. If you don't think you can wait the full 10 minutes, take a walk.

4. **Distance** yourself, physically, from the temptation. Walk out of the house, if you have to. Put some space between you and the food.

5. **Decide** how you will handle the craving: Will you give in or walk away? Sometimes, it's okay to give in. If you can *consciously* decide that yes, you really do want it, allow yourself one serving—and enjoy it thoroughly.

✔ **How's It Going?**
If you've made any poor food choices, were you able to get immediately back on track?

MIDDAY CRAVINGS: EAT RIGHT, BE READY

By far the greatest number of cravings occurs late in the day, from 3 to about 6 p.m. That's when your blood glucose drops, making your eyelids droop and igniting your desire to eat. During the dreaded midafternoon slump, all it takes is a cue—a co-worker's candy dish, for example—to find yourself drifting to the vending machine, or the coffee shop downstairs, for a little fat- and sugar-fueled "motivation."

Forewarned is forearmed: If you know a food craving will strike, you can outwit it, rather than surrender to it.

One of the best ways to head off midafternoon cravings is to defeat them in the morning—with a protein-packed breakfast. In a study conducted at the University of Connecticut, people who ate eggs rather than a bagel in the morning consumed fewer calories all day and felt satisfied longer. And people who downed 2½ cups of fat-free milk with their breakfast reported feeling less hungry and consumed fewer calories at lunch, according to a study in the *American Journal of Clinical Nutrition*. I don't think you have to drink that much with a meal—a cup will likely work just fine—but you see the importance of starting the day off right.

Eat a healthy lunch, too. You'll be less likely

to experience a craving for sweets if you consume enough calories at lunch, and if your lunch contains adequate amounts of protein.

Another tactic: Know your unique craving time (3:30 p.m.? during the drive home?) and preempt the craving. The idea is, if you have a bit of what you crave before the craving hits, you're less likely to lust for it. For example, if you tend to reach for sweets in the midafternoon, have a small square of chocolate at lunch. If you tend to crave salt at this time, add a pickle to your lunch. Just don't eat it alone, because if you have it as a snack you will still be hungry.

Bring your own healthy snack to work, if possible. Bashi, thirty-three, used to battle midafternoon cravings, usually for sweets. Now her cravings are gone and she lost forty-seven pounds over eighteen months, which she's kept off for a year. "These days, if I have something sweet, it leaves me unsatisfied ninety-five percent of the time," she says. "Now, I'll usually go for a piece of fruit with nuts or baby carrots with hummus to hold me until dinner."

I can't stress enough that you need to prepare for midafternoon cravings. You wouldn't march to battle without ammunition, would you? Then don't head into your prime craving time without healthy snack alternatives. Still, I get patients who never tire of telling me why they weren't prepared.

I always crave something sweet around 4 p.m. I know I should be prepared, but I always forget to bring a snack from home.

Small Change Solution: Remember, the best way to defeat cravings is to nip them in the bud! If you can remember that you're always hungry at 4 p.m., then you can remember to bring a healthy snack from home—or buy one on your way to work or when you pick up breakfast or lunch. Bringing healthy snacks with you is a habit that you cultivate. So tonight, before you go to bed, place an apple or pear with a snack-size baggie of nuts next to your keys. Or place a sticky note on your bathroom mirror, reminding you to grab a low-fat yogurt or cottage cheese from your refrigerator to keep in the office refrigerator.

I bring a healthy snack every day to work and eat it around 3 p.m. But it never fails that by 5 p.m., I crave something salty! That's when I make my way to the office vending machine for a bag of chips.

Small Change Solution: Perhaps you're eating lunch too early. If you know you have cravings at around 5 p.m., you might try rescheduling your meals to accommodate them. For example, if you usually eat lunch at noon and your snack at 3 p.m., try moving lunch to 1 p.m. and your snack to 4:30 p.m. Your new meal schedule might just preempt your craving. Also, if you crave salt, it's OK to allow yourself a serving of baked chips or pita crisps. But team your salty snack with satisfying protein, such as ½ ounce of nuts, a serving of low-fat yogurt, or even a glass of low-fat milk. Or if you have no choice in what time you eat lunch, try a pickle at 3 p.m. One salty pickle just might do the trick.

Midafternoon Cravings Options

If you crave *sweet*, try:

- a piece of fruit with ½ ounce of nuts
- 1 cup plain low-fat yogurt with fresh berries/1 tablespoon jam or a serving of low-fat flavored yogurt
- ½ cup low-fat cottage cheese with fresh or frozen berries
- a "tall" decaf soy latte

If you crave *chocolate* particularly, try:

- 8 ounces low-fat chocolate milk

- 8 ounces hot chocolate made with low-fat milk

- 8 ounces chocolate soy beverage

If you crave *salt*, try:

- a serving of soy crisps

- ½ cup low-fat cottage cheese

- 1 cup miso soup

- 1 ounce roasted edamame or salted nuts

- ½ cup salted boiled edamame

Small Change Midday Cravings Tips

1. Always eat a protein-packed breakfast and lunch to help suppress cravings that may occur later.

2. Identify your craving—whether it's for salt or sugar, creamy or crunchy—and satisfy it appropriately.

3. Think of your midday craving as an opportunity to enjoy a healthy afternoon snack.

4. Be prepared. Bring a well-balanced snack to work so you don't have to hit the vending machines or the office candy jar.

5. Buy snack foods that are prepackaged in single-serving sizes so you won't be tempted to overeat.

NIGHT CRAVINGS: EAT LATER, KEEP BUSY, STAY STRONG

If you're often plagued with cravings late at night—and many people are—consider your eating habits.

- Are you eating enough calories at each meal?

- Are you eating enough fiber-rich fruits and veggies each day?

- Are you getting enough protein and fat at each meal?

- Are you eating your two snacks a day?

If you answered yes to all four questions, your cravings are likely all in your head. That may sound harsh, but there it is: If you're eating enough, and you're also consuming enough fat and protein, it is unlikely that you are experiencing true physical hunger. What you may be experiencing: stress or boredom. Or perhaps you're simply used to eating what you want at night. So the best "prescription" for late-night cravings is to eat enough—and well—during the day. If you already do that, it's time to try a few time-tested tactics to beat the late-night munchies.

One simple fix: If you typically eat dinner early—say, by 6 or 6:30 p.m.—but stay up until midnight or later, you might push your dinner back to 8 or 8:30. That way, you'll be safely in bed before late-night cravings kick in. The solution sounds almost too simple, but it works.

Another way to head off late-night cravings is to plan a healthy evening snack, and enjoy it after 9 p.m. You don't need to pair your evening snack with protein, since you'll be in bed in a few hours and won't need the snack to hold you over until your next meal.

Evening Cravings Options

If you crave *sweet*, try:

- a piece of fruit

- sugar-free ice pops*

- diet gelatin*

---

* Feel free to have more than one serving, but try not to have more than two. Although these snacks are very low calorie, you're not dealing with the *behavior* of nighttime eating.

If you crave *chocolate*, try:

- 8 ounces hot chocolate made with low-fat milk

- 8 ounces low-fat chocolate milk

- 8 ounces chocolate soy beverage

- 1 low-fat frozen fudge bar

- 1 serving low-fat chocolate pudding

If you crave *salt*, try:

- 3 cups air-popped popcorn with spray butter and a dash of salt

- 1 serving pretzels (sticks, twists, or rods, not the big sourdough kind)

- ½ ounce nuts (less than a serving, so you don't consume too many calories before bed)

If you choose to have a snack, enjoy it, and then make the kitchen off-limits. Instead of wandering in and out of the kitchen, turn your attention to a hobby or activity you enjoy. Knit, read, meditate, paint—any activity that keeps your mind off food and your hands busy. Try and limit late-night TV watching since it doesn't keep your hands busy (except for channel surfing), and some commercials may only increase your cravings. A good idea is to have a DVR and tape your TV programs so you can skip commercials altogether.

Sometimes, however, you simply have to "urge surf," like my patient Meredith, twenty-eight. "My worst cravings—especially for salty foods, like chips—hit in the evening after dinner and before bed," she confessed. Sometimes, she'll opt for a serving of sliced chicken or a 100-calorie package of chips, But her cravings don't always fade. "It can be a struggle to not go out and buy a bigger bag of chips, or eat only one hundred-calorie bag," she said. "But I've learned that, more often than not, my cravings don't stem from hunger, but from other emotions, including boredom. I try to let those feelings pass and not give in to them."

I hear many excuses for caving in to unhealthy nighttime cravings. The ones below are the most common:

My husband loves ice cream. Unfortunately, so do I. Although I buy it for him, and can leave it alone during the day, I always weaken at night.

Small Change Solution: If you lived alone, I'd tell you not to buy the ice cream in the first place—you can't eat what you don't have in the house! But husbands (or wives) do love their ice cream, and wives (or husbands) aren't made of stone . . . and I suspect you feel a bit deprived when you watch your husband enjoy his favorite flavor. And feelings of deprivation breed cravings.

So here's a simple solution: Buy a low-calorie frozen dessert for yourself. There are lots to choose from, including low-fat ice cream sandwiches, low-fat or sugar-free frozen yogurt, and yummy sugar-free pops. So when your husband enjoys his "treat," you don't feel left out.

I don't eat much during the day because I know I will eat a lot after dinner. This way I can still enjoy my late-night snacks and not feel guilty about overeating.

Small Change Solution: What you describe is very much a "what came first, the chicken or the egg?" situation. In other words, I think you overeat at night *because* you don't eat much during the day—and while you may think you are saving calories, you end up consuming more in the long run. Get on a healthy schedule (Small Change 1) and see if that doesn't stop your nighttime cravings. Who says you can't enjoy some of your late-night snacks during the day?

Small Change Evening Cravings Tips

1. Make sure you consume enough calories, fiber, and protein at dinner.

2. If you're a night owl, eat dinner no earlier than 7 p.m.

3. Establish a "kitchen closed" policy after dinner. Put a sticky note on the fridge to remind you.

4. Brush your teeth soon after dinner.

5. If you must keep your hands busy after dinner, turn to a hobby or activity you enjoy that does not involve food.

IF YOU OVERINDULGE, GET BACK ON TRACK

Every once in a while, I have to console a client who overindulges. He or she woke up stuffed the morning after a party, or on a Monday after a weekend of pancake breakfasts and an all-you-can-eat buffet, feeling guilty and discouraged (not to mention bloated). But I don't let my clients wallow in that negativity. Everyone overindulges at times, and chances are, you will, too. The key is how you rebound from it.

First things first: Don't beat yourself up. While it's important to admit that you overdid it, it's equally important to forgive yourself and move on. If you don't, it's all too easy to let one slip derail all your hard work.

Step back from the scale, too. Try to relax about whether you've regained weight. It is unlikely that one off day will undo weeks or months of careful, healthy eating. Even if you gain a pound or two, it's likely just water weight from salt.

Don't be surprised if you wake up hungry the morning after a day of overeating. That's not unusual. Or some of my patients tell me that they are still full when they wake up. If either happens, maintain your usual nutritious morning meal (don't forget the protein). Starving yourself out of guilt or not eating because you don't yet have an appetite will only set you up for overeating later in the day, and you don't want to go there. After breakfast, resume your healthy eating plan for the rest of the day.

The day after overindulging, drink more water than usual, to help flush out salt. Resume your Healthy Plate method—remember, go heavy on the fruits and veggies—and get out for a brisk walk or to the gym.

While I tell my patients that it's fine to "indulge"

every once in a while, some still do it all too often. Do their rationalizations sound like yours?

It's always the same thing—I do well for a few weeks, and then I blow it. I just don't have any willpower, I guess.

Small Change Solution: While willpower can help you stick to a healthy eating plan, don't be so hard on yourself. You didn't blow anything. No one eats perfectly all the time. In fact, I encourage my patients to focus not on perfection, but on eating healthy 80 percent of the time. If you happen to make poor choices, what's important is to let it go and get right back on track, so one slip doesn't sabotage all your hard work.

What's the use? I've already blown it—might as well have the rest of these cookies.

Small Change Solution: As I said above, you didn't blow anything. It's the all-or-nothing thinking that can really sabotage you. Two cookies fit into a healthy eating plan—an entire box doesn't. So don't deprive yourself of the foods you love; you'll set yourself up to overdo it. Instead of thinking cookies are off-limits entirely, try accepting that two small cookies can fit in and that you can enjoy them.

Small Change Overindulgence Tips

1. Ditch the guilt—it's useless and may delay your ability to get back on track.

2. Eat normally at your next meal—don't skip it.

3. Get some exercise as soon as possible to help boost your mood.

4. Reflect on your overindulgence. You may learn something to head off the next one.

5. Call a supportive friend and talk about "falling off the wagon." A sympathetic ear can help you regroup and refire your motivation.

WHAT TO EAT "THE DAY AFTER"

What should you eat to regain control after a day of overindulging? Pretty much the same healthy-eating plan you follow each day, with a few targeted changes.

Eat a smaller breakfast if you wish (but you don't have to), and opt for either the following suggested snack ideas or the healthy snack you eat every day to keep cravings at bay. You might want to skip alcohol, too, since it can reduce your inhibitions and lead to overeating. Don't forget the fluids either.

Drinking plenty of water, sparkling water, or seltzer (sodium-free) can reduce day-after bloating.

If you're not hungry, eat the following breakfast:

   1 slice whole-wheat toast

   1 tablespoon of natural peanut butter topped with ½ sliced banana

If you have your regular morning appetite, eat the following breakfast:

   1 egg, cooked without fat (e.g., hard-boiled, poached)

   Cooked oatmeal, made with ½ cup dry oats and 1 cup nonfat or 1 percent milk (stir in 1 tablespoon ground flax and sprinkle with cinnamon)

   4 ounces orange juice mixed with 4 ounces seltzer (for a serving of fruit plus extra fluids)

Midmorning snack

   1 cup plain nonfat or low-fat yogurt

   1 cup berries

   (If you're truly not hungry, you may eat half.)

Lunch

1½ cups mixed greens topped with ½ cup chickpeas, ¼ avocado, sliced tomato, onion, cucumbers, carrots (or other raw veggies of your choice), and 3 ounces grilled chicken

2 tablespoons low-fat salad dressing

8 ounces nonfat milk

Afternoon snack

½ ounce nuts (the amount that would fill half a shot glass)

1 piece fruit

(Or, enjoy the healthy snack that best eases your midafternoon cravings.)

Dinner

1 cup mixed greens, topped with your choice of raw veggies

2 tablespoons low-fat salad dressing

3 ounces broiled salmon

1 cup steamed broccoli

½ cup quinoa

Evening snack

1 cup berries

(Or, enjoy the healthy snack that best eases your evening cravings.)

ARE YOU READY TO MOVE ON?

Hopefully, you now know that cravings don't have to blindside you if you anticipate and plan for them. Eating healthy, balanced meals, eating enough during the day, and keeping healthy snacks at the ready—and yes, even satisfying them once in a while—can tame even the strongest craving, no matter when it occurs. Take the Small Change Success Test below to see if you are ready to move on to the next Small Change.

Small Change Success Test

1. Do you use the HALT technique any time you experience cravings?

2. Do you plan for cravings, either by bringing your own healthy snack with you or buying one?

3. Do you choose low-calorie alternatives to your craved foods?

---

4. Do you eat enough during the day, and keep busy at night, to vanquish late-night cravings?

5. If you've overindulged, did you ditch the guilt and get back on track immediately?

If you answered yes to no more than three of the items on this chapter's Small Change Success Test, go back to the plan and keep plugging away at the Small Changes that challenge you, one at a time. It may take you a while to work your way through the list, but if my patients can do it, so can you!

If you've answered yes to at least four questions, congratulations. It's time to tackle another Small Change.

▼▲▼▲▼▲▼▲▼

Share Food and Good Times with Advance Planning— and Without Guilt

We all celebrate special occasions by dining out or going to parties, or by having "special" foods in the house at certain times of the year. We travel. We go to lunch with friends. We have business events. We eat to be social. Too often we sabotage our good habits in these situations. So many of my patients gain weight over the holidays or complain that their busy social calendar is what causes their eating to get out of control. But it's possible to be sociable and thin for life.

There are several reasons that special events can be hard to navigate when you're on a weight loss plan. First, you don't have established patterns of eating in these circumstances—every occasion offers different temptations. For example, at a wedding, there's the cake. On vacation, there may be day after day of open buffet. At a holiday office party, there are the five different kinds of hors d'oeuvres. Then there's the social component. If you're in a situation where you don't know many people, it can be easier to hang out by the food than to make small talk with strangers. Finally, it can be difficult to resist the celebratory nature of these events. Good food and good times go together, right?

Of course they do. But you've worked so hard to come this far. Why turn a happy occasion into cause for regret by sabotaging your eating plan? While you may decide to relax your plan just a bit, giving yourself permission to enjoy your favorite foods in sensible portions, it makes sense to stay on track as closely as you can. This is not to deprive yourself, but to learn to use all the Small Changes that we've discussed so far, and to learn to eat in a way that's doable for life. That's what this chapter is all about—and fortunately, you can let the good times roll, without sabotaging all your hard work.

BEFORE YOU PARTY, PLAN

To navigate the event with your healthy diet intact, you need a plan. Devising one that's tailored to the social occasion, and then sticking to it, will help you handle a day (or night) of eating and drinking.

Your strategy begins even before the event does.

1. **On the day of the celebration, eat normally before you go.** *Please* don't skip breakfast and/or lunch so you can "spend" those calories at the event. By party time, you'll be tired, irritable, and primed to eat everything in arm's length.

   On the other hand, eating sensibly will take the edge off your appetite and arm you with the restraint you'll need. If possible, work out the day of your event, too. For some reason, when you hit the gym, or take your daily brisk walk, it reinforces your commitment to a healthy lifestyle, which in turn lessens the odds of overindulging.

2. **Snack before you go.** A snack that pairs carbs and protein—say, a piece of string cheese and an apple, or a serving of low-fat cottage cheese and a serving of cut-up fruit—will take the edge off your hunger and help you withstand cravings, so you'll make smarter decisions when you face the menu, buffet table, or dessert cart.

3. **Get back on track immediately after the event.**
   While you should strive to follow your eating
   plan as closely as possible, it's understandable
   if you eat a little more than you'd planned at
   a wedding or on vacation. If you overindulge,
   get over the guilt—and right back on your
   healthy plan.

If you drink alcohol, you'll also need to have a
drinking plan. Alcohol lowers inhibitions, raising
the odds that you'll gobble hors d'oeuvres or succumb to salt or sugar cravings. To avoid overindulging, set a one- or two-drink limit, then decide
when you'll have it. If you'll be at a cocktail party,
you may choose to have your drinks shortly after
you arrive. If you're attending a wedding recep-
tion, you might have one when you arrive, and
another for the toast. Opt for a low-calorie libation
(you'll find several smart choices in Small Change
3) and stick to water, seltzer, or sparkling water the
rest of the time.

Even the best-laid plans can go awry, of course. If
you go overboard, no worries—as the saying goes,
what happens in Vegas stays in Vegas. Just get back
on track immediately (Small Change 8).

Your Small Change Plan

1. Dine out, rather than pig out.

2. Celebrate the event, not the food.

3. Treat "the holidays" as one day, not one month.

4. Take a vacation from work, not from eating smart.

RESTAURANT DINING: ENJOY
WITHOUT GAINING WEIGHT

Here's a bold statement for you: You could eat every one of your meals at a restaurant every day for a full year and still maintain or lose weight—if you made smart choices.

These days, you just can't use dining out as an excuse to eat poorly. Even national chain restaurants offer healthy choices alongside their fat and sugar bombs, and you can order a salad, broiled fish or chicken, and fruit for dessert almost anywhere, even if you're facing down an all-you-can-eat buffet at a hotel on vacation or on a cruise.

Am I saying you *should* eat like a Spartan at a celebration or on vacation? No. Am I saying that you can stick to your normal, well-balanced, healthy eating plan if you choose to? Absolutely. The choice is yours. That said, there are plenty of ways you can enjoy a dinner out or the food on your vacation. Small changes, simple steps.

I've already shot down the "don't eat all day so I can pig out at night" strategy—it will definitely backfire, because you will be so hungry by the time you sit down that you will likely overeat. But a realistic Small Change is to skip the bread typically offered before the meal. Unless it's to die for, it's not worth eating. What if it's heavenly? Do what my patient Sara, twenty-seven, does. "When I'm out to dinner, it's either bread or wine—not both," she said. "If the bread is amazing, I'll have one small piece but back off on the wine and see if I can substitute the starch on my main entrée for veggies." If the people you're dining with want the bread (even if it's so-so), position the bread basket as far away from you as possible.

Read the menu very carefully. In fact, see if you can read it online *before* you go. Many restaurants put their menus online these days, so you can "order" before you even step foot in the place. Don't be afraid to ask exactly how a meal is prepared. It's okay to say, "Could you prepare the fish with olive oil instead of butter?" or, "Could I have a double order of broccoli instead of the rice pilaf?" If you're at an all-you-can-eat buffet, examine every offering first, and then decide what you will have. If you don't trust yourself to control your portions or eat the healthiest offerings, skip the buffet and order from the menu.

Seems like my patients are dining out more than ever. While many are getting the hang of it nicely, a few still have excuses for why they didn't choose wisely:

I often go out to dinner with clients and don't get to choose the place. We never go to a fish restaurant.

Small Change Solution: You can't blame restaurants—or your clients—for making poor choices or overeating. These days, most establishments offer a few healthy alternatives for their health-conscious patrons, including grilled chicken, or fish (even at steakhouses), salad, veggies, and fruit. Even ethnic cuisines have at least a few lighter dishes. All you need to do—at any restaurant—is follow the Healthy Plate method, watch your portions, order your entrée "naked" (prepared without high-fat ingredients like butter or cream), skip the bread, and order sauces on the side. Okay, you may not eat perfectly. But you *can* take steps to ensure that what goes on your plate doesn't end up around your waistline.

I am single and frequently go to dinner on dates and with friends. I don't want to appear picky, so I eat a lot of things I know I shouldn't.

Small Change Solution: Being a health-conscious eater doesn't mean you are picky. I always tell my patients to be a leader, not a follower. Order first, and then encourage your friends to order a healthy meal that includes items such as a salad, vegetable-based soup, shrimp cocktail, veggies, and (grilled) fish or chicken. Just ask the waiter nicely and don't make a scene. Knowing what is good for you and your body is a positive thing. Be proud of it.

Small Change Dining-Out Tips

1. Skip the bread.

2. Start with a salad.

3. Read the menu carefully, looking for dishes prepared "broiled," "grilled," "steamed," and "sautéed," rather than "fried," "crispy," or "creamy."

4. Don't be afraid to ask questions about how a dish is prepared.

5. Order all sauces and dressings—including salad dressing—on the side.

6. Request a veggie instead of fries or other high-calorie sides (pay extra if you have to).

7. More often than not, opt for broiled fish or roasted, broiled, or grilled chicken without skin.

8. If you know the restaurant serves large portions, split an entrée with a friend or have two appetizers instead of an entrée.

9. If you're served a huge portion, eat half and take the other half home in a doggie bag for the next day.

10. If you want dessert, split one with others in your party (the more forks, the better!).

FIND HEALTHY CHOICES ON ANY MENU

Whether you're dining with friends or family, or doing a business lunch or dinner, there's no need to get sideways on your healthy eating—even if you're dining at a steakhouse or an ethnic eatery. Below you'll find some of the healthiest entrées, along with those to pass up. Start with a salad and dressing on the side, skip the bread, and watch your portions and alcoholic beverages, and you'll do fine.

Chinese

Pass up egg rolls, spareribs, fried dumplings, pork lo mein, fried rice, moo shu, General Tso's chicken, sweet-and-sour pork, wonton soup.

Opt for steamed or stir-fried seafood, chicken, bean curd or vegetable dishes, egg drop soup; rice (½ cup; request brown rice, if available).

French

Pass up quiche, pommes frites (French fries), cordon bleu, croissant, pate, foie gras, sausage, escargot, any dish (including soups) made with cream or cheese.

Opt for salad with vinaigrette dressing, bouillabaisse, roasted poultry, braised meat, mussels, oysters, ratatouille, steamed or grilled vegetables.

Indian

Pass up any dish with *paneer* (Indian cheese), korma sauce (made with cream) or coconut, any dish with *malai* (cream) or *makhani* (with butter).

Opt for chicken or shrimp Tandoori, vegetable

curries, vegetarian dishes cooked with spices but without clarified butter (ghee), naan (half a small).

Italian

Pass up garlic bread, meat sauces (like Bolognese), cheesy sauces (like alfredo), fried calamari, pastas stuffed with cheese, veal/chicken or eggplant Parmesan.

Opt for light sauces, like marinara, primavera, clam, or marsala (wine, mushrooms, beef stock), *branzino* (sea bass), mussels *fra diavolo*.

Japanese

Pass up any kind of tempura, fried *gyoza* (the Japanese version of Chinese pot stickers) or fried wonton, *agedashi* tofu (deep-fried tofu), *nikuitame* (stir-fried pork), specialty rolls (may have more ingredients than basic rolls).

Opt for seaweed salad, miso soup, broiled sea bass (or any broiled fish), yakitori (grilled chicken), steamed *gyoza*, sushi, nigiri, sashimi, edamame, *ohitashi* (steamed spinach).

Mediterranean/Middle Eastern

Pass up moussaka, gyros, falafel, baklava (a Greek pastry).

Opt for Greek salad, shish kabob, souvlaki

(chicken, not lamb), fish cooked in tomatoes (or any fish dish), hummus or baba ganoush (two tablespoons), pita bread (one small), tabouleh.

Mexican

Pass up chips, fried tacos, refried beans, quesadillas, chimichangas, enchiladas, beef burritos.

Opt for black beans, black-bean soup, grilled shrimp, grilled chicken or fish, chicken or shrimp fajitas.

Steakhouse

Pass up fried appetizers, creamy soups, ribs, loaded baked potato, porterhouse steak, rib eye, onion rings, French fries.

Opt for side salad, steamed veggies, baked potato (half; no butter or sour cream); grilled chicken, London broil, filet mignon, flank steak, sirloin tip, tenderloin, seafood, peel-'n'-eat shrimp, oysters on the half shell.

Thai

Pass up fried spring rolls, *tom ka gai* (coconut chicken soup), duck.

Opt for steamed spring rolls, hot-and-sour soup, pad Thai (stir-fried noodles), vegetable stir-fries, sticky rice (½ cup).

✔ *How's It Going?*

Are you getting enough sleep every night, so you're less likely to make poor food choices the next day?

CELEBRATE THE EVENT, NOT THE FOOD

Whether you're headed to a wedding, birthday, graduation party, or a Super Bowl get-together, keep one thing in mind: The best part of a party isn't the food, but the company. At least, that's the way it should be!

Before you step out the door, commit to socializing. If you're going to a wedding, make sure to get out on the dance floor. Cocktail party? Strike up a conversation with a person you don't know but who looks interesting. (Hint: Ask them a lot of questions—that's what I do, and it works beautifully.) Family reunion? Catch up with old friends or relatives you haven't seen in years, or ever. If you approach your gathering with a mission—to socialize—food will assume its rightful place at the gathering: a pleasure, but not the star attraction.

Of course, food will be there, and there's nothing wrong with enjoying it—in sensible amounts. A great, all-purpose rule is, position yourself as far away from the food as possible. But there are other strategies, too—pick one that suits the occasion. For example, if you've been invited to an evening cocktail party where hors d'oeuvres will be served, bring a clutch purse. As you chat and mingle with the guests, hold your glass in one hand, and your bag in the other. You won't be able to hold a plate. Or if you're attending a function with a buffet, peruse the food table first—without a plate in your hand—and *then* go back and choose healthy items, rather than pile your plate high.

If you're invited to a party at someone's home and want to make sure there will be something that fits into your healthy eating plan, volunteer to bring a fruit salad, hummus-and-raw-veggie plate, or a covered dish made with low-fat ingredients. Problem solved—for you and, I'm betting, at least a few of the other guests.

If you'll be attending a gathering where the food is out for the duration, don't pick up a plate until you feel true, physical hunger. If you've had a snack before the party, you'll know. When you get hungry, use the buffet strategy—do a "look-see" at the food table and decide what you'll have.

When you've decided, make up one plate, using the Healthy Plate method as much as possible.

If there's salad or other veggies prepared without high-fat ingredients (fresh green beans, zucchini, broccoli), you're in luck. Add a serving of meat, poultry, or fish without sauce and maybe a tiny taste of something you truly love, so you won't feel deprived. Maybe you give up the potato salad to have a small brownie; maybe you have a green salad and a small piece of lasagna. The point is, choose wisely so you can have a serving of a food you truly love.

Then, enjoy every bite of what you choose. Try to make your meal last thirty minutes (chat while you eat and sip your wine, water, or sparkling water), and stop when you are full.

If you're at a wedding, there's plenty of time to socialize and not focus just on the food. And when the food comes, enjoy it, leaving the fattiest part of your meal on your plate if you know no matter what you will eat the wedding cake or by savoring just a bite of cake if you choose to eat your full meal.

Like everyone else, my patients love to celebrate. A few, however, have reasons for why things might not go so well:

During football season I watch the games with my boyfriend and his friends. It's fun,

but I always drink too much beer and eat too much—chips, chicken wings, mozzarella sticks. I don't want to stay home, but I can't seem to lose weight when I go.

Small Change Solution: Quite the dilemma, trying to be one of the guys. Problem is the "guys" don't realize they shouldn't overeat either. I tell my patients that when they watch sports, to appreciate the stamina that goes into the athletes' performances. If they were eating like crap, too, the game wouldn't be worth watching!

If that isn't enough motivation, have a healthy, well-balanced snack before you go, or bring your own low-cal munchies from home, like raw sliced veggies with low-fat dip, air-popped popcorn, or a Tupperware container of strawberries. If you're going to drink, stick to light beer—bring your own if you have to, and nurse those one or two bottles. Then stick to water or diet soda and enjoy the game!

Every week, it seems, there's another office birthday to celebrate . . . and another cake to eat. Sometimes I can resist it at the party, but then it sits in the break room all day and come 4 p.m., it's hard to resist!

Small Change Solution: Office birthday celebrations aren't as tricky as they seem. At the party, accept the slice of cake you're offered, and hold it as you chat with your colleagues. You can even eat it, if you work in an office that celebrates all birthdays once a month. Just have a small slice. You may just decide to pass on it one day—especially if your business clothing is feeling deliciously loose. And if you have your healthy snacks with you, I bet that cake won't look so tempting in the midafternoon.

Small Change Celebration Tips

1. Before you leave for your gathering, commit to focusing on socializing, rather than eating.

2. Position yourself away from where the hors d'oeuvres are set up.

3. Pass on any fried or high-fat hors d'oeuvres, i.e., pigs in a blanket.

4. Peruse the buffet table before filling your plate.

5. If you are not given an option for your entrée and it is high in fat/calories, try to eat only half.

6. Pass on the bread basket.

7. Limit alcohol intake to two drinks. Sip seltzer in between.

8. Have one slice of celebratory cake, but don't finish it.

9. If there is a dance floor, get on it.

10. If your host is offering any high-calorie and fat-laden leftovers (i.e., cake) to go, kindly decline.

IT'S THE HOLI*DAY*, NOT THE HOLI*WEEK* OR MONTH

Thanksgiving, Christmas, or Hanukkah, Easter, Independence Day . . . the holidays bring family and friends together to celebrate and spread good cheer. They also bring lots of opportunities for social eating and drinking. Even so, it's possible to enjoy your holiday favorites—in sensible portions— without packing on the pounds. To do that, follow the three-part default strategy at the beginning of the chapter: eat normally the day of the event, snack before it occurs, and get back to your normal eating immediately. Watch your alcohol intake, too.

Here's a welcome gift. I don't care what you eat on Thanksgiving, or Christmas, or Easter. If you want to overeat, go for it. I even tell my patients they don't have to food journal for the day. But after that one day, that's it. That's the condition. No repeat performances. Don't take leftovers home with you. If you're the one doing the cooking, buy lots of food-storage containers with lids, and send everyone home with food.

If your holidays are not filled with only one meal but many—cocktail parties, business celebrations, and the like—then plan your eating strategy well in advance. For example, if you have one Thanksgiving dinner at your parents' house and another the next day at your in-laws', consider what and how much you will eat at each dinner.

You might decide, for example, to have your blowout at your parents' dinner and to eat lightly at your in-laws', but have a slice of her special pumpkin pie or her killer mashed potatoes. You don't want to insult anyone by not eating, so eat. Just have small portions. If they offer you seconds, do not say, "I'm on a diet." You are not dieting. You're eating healthfully, which includes watching your portion sizes. So work on your nicest, "No thanks. It's all so delicious, but I'm stuffed!"

If you are the one doing the cooking, make those traditional favorites your family has come to expect and that you enjoy making. Simply add some healthy alternatives, like a salad or veggies, prepared without fat. Or modify your recipes. Prepare them with low-fat ingredients and serve sauces on the side. Chances are, no one will notice. If you're not cooking, offer to bring those healthy alternatives to the feast. People will eat them. And if they don't, so what? You will, and that's what counts.

If you're hosting the event, why not add fun and games to the day? It's a great way to break the tradition of dozing on the couch, uncomfortably stuffed, after the meal. If you typically host Thanksgiving dinner, propose a game of touch football; at Christmas, skate, sled, or build a group snowman. For a July Fourth celebration, set up the badminton net or break out the horseshoes or croquet set. Or simply go for a long walk. For indoor fun, there's Pictionary or charades. (My family loves a good game of Ping-Pong!) While food is always part of the holidays, so is family—and when food shares the spotlight, instead of commanding it, you may have more fun than you ever imagined.

Holidays can be a happy time but many of my patients complain of stress caused by spending time with family (or not). They also have stress around their holiday eating. These are some of the excuses I hear:

My family goes to my parents' house for Thanksgiving, and every year my mother makes her "special" apple pie for me because "I love it." I do, but don't want to get off track with my new eating habits.

Small Change Solution: Go ahead and have that slice. One slice, on the small side. You can, and still stay on track. Just don't take the leftover pie home, even if she insists. If she insists, explain to your mother that eating pie at this moment of your life is difficult for you and that you need to abstain. I am sure your mother is baking out of love for you, and hopefully she can respect your decision.

There are so many festivities around the holidays—and food at every one. I'm also constantly gifted with cookies and candy. I eat them because, well, they're gifts. I don't want to come off like Scrooge.

Small Change Solution: Sounds like you might be confusing the food at these celebrations with the celebration itself. Thanksgiving, Christmas, and New Year's Eve add up to three days, not six weeks. So enjoy whatever you like *on those three days*. Between those days, stick to your healthy-eating plan using the suggestions in this change. When you're given cookies and candy, thank the giver, then give them to your doorman, postman, or next-door neighbor.

Small Change Holiday Tips

1. If you love it, eat it—for one day only.

2. Follow the strategies on pages 236–237 for cocktail parties, buffets, and alcohol intake.

3. If you're hosting, offer lower-calorie alternatives.

4. If you're a guest, bring those alternatives with you.

5. Send guests home with leftovers.

6. If you are a guest, refuse leftovers—nicely.

7. Enjoy your favorite dish, but don't take seconds.

8. If you don't love it, don't eat it.

9. If you opt for dessert, choose one, and have one serving.

10. Add (active) fun and games to the event, or indoor parlor games.

ON THE ROAD AGAIN . . .

Travel frequently on business? Just because you're eating away from home doesn't mean you can't eat like you *are* at home. These tips are just for you.

- Nowadays, most airports offer healthier choices. Make them yours.

- Buy water at the airport. Air travel is dehydrating.

- If your hotel room has a minibar (which will be packed with junk food and alcohol), refuse the key.

- If possible, book a hotel that has a gym. If you can't, pack resistance bands and a yoga mat, so you can do a quick workout in your room, or pack sneakers and go for a walk or run before or after your meetings.

- If you'll be going straight to a business dinner from meetings, bring a healthy snack, like nuts or a granola-type bar to keep midafternoon cravings at bay.

TAKE A VACATION FROM WORK, NOT HEALTHY EATING

Ah, vacation. Sunning on the beach or on the deck of a cruise ship. Taking in a show at a casino or a theme park with the kids. Eating way too much.

When you're on vacation, an irregular routine, free all-you-can-eat buffets, too many cocktails (piña coladas and strawberry daquiris), and free-flowing snacks (chips and salsa), or greasy fast-food lunches can make it all too easy to relax your healthy eating routine. But it is possible to stick to your plan—most of the time—and still enjoy yourself.

One of my patients, Carmela, forty-nine, has learned to be prepared when she travels. "By making sure I have snacks with me, I can stick to my regular eating plan," she said. Nor does she have a problem dining out when she travels. "Most restaurants offer healthy dishes, and they can be very good. Before, when I was a lot heavier, I'd order a pasta dish that came with a few pieces of protein. Now, I order a protein dish with a small portion of pasta." Strategies like these have helped her lose forty-two pounds and keep them off for three years.

Because vacation is a time to relax and kick back, many people delight in the convenience (and decadence) of room service and the minibar. However, these options can lead to vacation-induced weight gain. Be smart: Don't take the minibar key when you check into your hotel. If you decide to order room service, follow the same dining-out strategies. (I particularly love to order in breakfast—scrambled egg whites, hold the potatoes and toast, and a bowl of oatmeal.)

If your hotel offers a Continental breakfast, pass up the muffins and doughnuts and opt for the healthier fare, such as fruit and whole-grain cereals. If your hotel features a make-your-own omelet bar, enjoy egg white omelets stuffed with fresh veggies and a slice or two of whole-grain toast. And by the way, all-you-can-eat buffets, popular on cruise ships, are tempting, but there's no need to stuff yourself just because it's included.

If you know that your vacation condo or hotel room has a kitchenette with a microwave and refrigerator, go grocery shopping when you arrive. Stock your fridge with items for a healthy breakfast or lunch, save money (and your waistline), and dine out for dinners only.

If you're visiting attractions and exploring the area, pack a healthy snack—this might save you from grabbing a burger and fries, or pizza, when you or the kids get hungry. Better yet, before you embark on your day's activities, ask the concierge at the hotel for a suggestion on where to stop that might have healthier fare. Be adventurous and seek out local cuisine in the areas you are traveling. It's nice to sample a variety of in-season fruits, vegetables, and fresh-caught seafood that you may not get a chance to eat at home.

But if you do splurge, enjoy it! Remember, you are on vacation. But don't let it sabotage your successful weight loss to date. Simply try to eat healthier when you can for the rest of your trip, and most important, arrive home ready to get back on track.

I have patients who take active vacations (cycling, hiking) and who actually lose weight because they move more and nosh less. Others neither gain nor lose, which is fine. Yet others use their vacation as an excuse to eat, drink, and arrive home five pounds heavier. Their excuses sound like this:

I gain five pounds every time I go on vacation. Good food is part of the experience, right?

Small Change Solution: Absolutely. But you definitely don't have to gain weight. I tell my patients they don't have to lose weight while they are away, but that they shouldn't gain. But, in fact, some of my patients *lose* weight on vacation—they hike, walk, or bicycle, and make healthy choices and watch their portions most of the time. Some even find that they face fewer temptations on vacation—

no office candy jar, no ice cream in the freezer, and no chips from the corner deli.

Also, are your vacations active or do you lounge on the deck of a cruise ship or sit by a pool most of the time? Perhaps you could make your vacations more active, since you can't use the excuse that you're too busy working to exercise. Even if not, you *can* make a conscious decision before you leave that your R&R won't be all about food. Go ahead, enjoy an extra dessert or a few more cocktails than usual. But confine your blowout to one or two nights and eat well the rest of the time.

I spend my vacation time visiting my parents or siblings at their homes. I end up eating what's in their kitchen, and what they make for dinner. Unfortunately, they never eat veggies and cook rather unhealthily.

Small Change Solution: While it's a shame that your family members don't eat as healthfully as they could, enjoying their company doesn't have to mean diet disaster for you. Tag along when they go food shopping and buy the foods you typically eat for breakfast and lunch. At dinner, eat what they make, just watch your portions. About the veggies, don't stress. They'll be waiting for you when you get home.

Small Change Vacation Tips

1. Don't skip meals. Watch your portion sizes.

2. Refuse the minibar key.

3. Follow the dining-out tips at the beginning of this chapter.

4. Ask the concierge at your hotel if he or she can recommend restaurants that serve relatively healthy fare.

5. Try to limit yourself to two low-calorie alcoholic drinks per day.

6. If you're flying, pack healthy transportable snack foods like nuts and granola-type bars to eat on the plane and to have when you get to your destination.

7. If you're traveling by car, pack a cooler with healthy snacks such as yogurt, fruit, and string cheese.

8. If your hotel room has a kitchenette with a fridge, find a supermarket and purchase healthy snack foods and easy-to-fix breakfast items.

9. Pack your sneakers and get active! Use the hotel gym or pool.

10. Come home ready to resume your healthy-eating plan.

ARE YOU READY TO MOVE ON?

Chances are, you won't know whether you're ready to move on until you're invited to or host an event that tests you—the holidays, a wedding, your vacation, a dinner out with friends, or a birthday cake at the office. But when a social event finally does end up on your calendar, you'll be prepared! Or perhaps you've already navigated a social occasion or two. How did you do? Take the Small Change Success Test below to see if you are ready to move on to the next Small Change.

Small Change Success Test

1. Did you dine out, rather than pig out?

2. Did you celebrate the event, not the food?

3. Did you celebrate the holi*day*, rather than the holi*week* or month?

4. If you went on vacation, did you stick to healthy eating most of the time?

If you answered yes to no more than two of the items in this chapter's Small Change Success Test, don't stress—celebrations and social events challenge even the most health-conscious among us. You'll do better next time.

If you've answered yes to three or more questions, congratulations. It's time to tackle another Small Change!

▼▲▼▲▼▲▼▲▼

Get Moving

It's been said that exercise is like a savings account: The more you put in, the more you get back—with interest. It's hard to argue with that folksy wisdom. Exercise does benefit your body and mind in a multitude of ways. Just one brisk walk a day protects your health, boosts your mood, and generally improves the quality of your life.

So why do so many people hate exercise so much?

I've worked with hundreds of patients, and I think it comes down to this: Most people have a fixed idea of what exercise *should* be and think that it should be long, hard, boring, and sweaty. And it's true that exercise can be all those things—if you don't make an effort to change your thinking about it.

I promised you Small Changes that add up

to big weight loss. So I'm happy to tell you that the Small Changes I suggest in this chapter can net you impressive results. You will not only reap all those benefits I just mentioned but also lose weight more easily, and maybe bust through a plateau or two. It's not just me saying this. Study after study shows that regular exercise, teamed with a healthy diet, is the best way to lose weight and keep lost pounds lost. There's no better proof than a study that's been going on for over fifteen years now—the National Weight Control Registry (NWCR). Founded in 1994 by two university scientists—one from the University of Colorado and the other from the Medical School of Brown University—the NWCR's goal was to learn *exactly* how regular people lost weight and kept it off. (Anyone over the age of eighteen who has lost at least thirty pounds and maintained that loss for more than a year can enroll in the ongoing study.) Since then, more than five thousand people have enrolled—and shared their personal tips for weight loss success.

One thing 90 percent of them do is exercise. In fact, on average, NWCR enrollees get 60 minutes or more of moderate to high-intensity exercise a day. They love to walk—the walkers log five or six miles a day, on average.

Am I saying you have to do the same? No. But they're great role models, and these "losers" are the best evidence yet that if you want to lose weight, you've got to get, and keep, moving. In this chapter, I'll focus on four Small Changes that will help you shed those extra pounds and improve your health, to boot.

Your Small Change Plan

1. Make exercise time, playtime.

2. Start slowly, and be active five days a week.

3. Step it up!

4. Find your exercise *why*.

TURN "WORK" INTO PLAY

It's been said before, but it bears repeating: If you're going to exercise—and it's a good idea, for health as well as weight loss—then for goodness' sake, pick an activity you enjoy (see the appendix for plentiful ideas). There are as many types of exercise as there are ice-cream flavors, so there's no reason to settle for vanilla when what you really want is strawberry.

When you pick a physical activity you enjoy,

then you're not really "exercising." You're playing. Think outside the box and expand your definition of what exercise can be—gardening, boxing, cross-country skiing—and you may actually begin to look forward to "playtime." This was certainly true for me. Over the years, I've lifted weights, cycled, taken spinning and boot camp classes, played tennis, boxed, and goodness knows what else. But I finally found my thing: yoga, which I've stuck with for over ten years now.

As you ponder your options, be honest with yourself. Do you prefer working out indoors or outside? Do you want to work out solo or with a buddy or even a group? Is there a certain sport you like to play (or used to love)? Do you need a challenge, or a low-key activity? These questions can help you home in on the type of exercise you might enjoy—and stick to.

If you're bored with your current routine, either try something completely different or add a new challenge to what you're doing now. For example, if you're already doing yoga and find yourself a bit bored, try a type you don't usually do, like Vinyasa, Bikram, Ashtanga, Anasura, or Iyengar, to mix things up. If you walk or cycle, take a different route. If you're lifting weights in a gym, try some new machines. If your gym has a pool, maybe try a water-aerobics class or simply do laps. If you're sick of working out alone, ask a friend on a walking date or make exercise a family affair, going on family hikes, bicycle rides, or cross-country skiing expeditions. Join a softball league. Bowl. Play Ping-Pong. Go horseback riding. Play golf and carry your clubs. Take a dance class—salsa or swing dancing can offer a great aerobic workout.

In the end, approach exercise the way a ten-year-old might: What's exercise? I'm going to go sledding, or climb a tree, or see how fast I can run. Bring a bit of that carefree wonder into your workout and you're sure to enjoy yourself that much more.

Some of my patients still have a hard time accepting that working out can be fun and give me many reasons why they still don't like to exercise:

I tried yoga because so many of my friends love it, but I am just not flexible enough. When I take a class with them I struggle from beginning to end—not fun!

Small Change Solution: First, not being flexible isn't a reason not to do yoga. In fact, doing yoga will increase your flexibility! Second, are your friends in an advanced class? There are many different styles of yoga, and some of them, like Ashtanga, are more demanding than others. If they're in an advanced class, no wonder you're not having fun!

Yoga studios can have different approaches and every teacher within them a different style; it's important to find the one that best suits you. The best way to learn is to sign up for a beginner's class—and make sure you try a single class before giving your credit card over for a series. Once you've found the right class, give yourself time to learn proper alignment and the easier poses before you attempt the more challenging poses or yoga styles. So start gradually, be patient, and give yourself some time for your practice to grow. You may be surprised at how quickly you limber up—and how exhilarating this ancient discipline can be.

When I was younger, I was a jock—played field hockey, softball, and basketball. But I'm too old to play a sport now.

Small Change Solution: Thinking inside the box, are you? Who says you still can't play sports? There are plenty of "master's leagues" for former jocks. If you played a particularly demanding sport, like football or field hockey, you might decide to join a volleyball or softball team instead, but you're still getting your exercise and—most important—reliving the joy of moving your body and the spirit of competition. Of course, you may want to see your doctor for a checkup, then begin a light training regimen before you join a master's league. This will help you avoid injury and ensure that you have just as good a time playing now as you did in high school.

> ### Small Change Make-Exercise-Fun Tips
>
> 1. When deciding on an exercise routine, think outside the box.
>
> 2. Approach exercise the way a child would— what would be *fun*?
>
> 3. Try an activity that's always intrigued you— fencing, cardio kickboxing, rock climbing.
>
> 4. Join a local walking or hiking group. You'll gain companionship as you burn calories.
>
> 5. If you dislike gyms, work out at home. Amass a library of fitness DVDs and podcasts or turn on a fitness channel on TV.

A WORD TO THE GYM-SHY

Many of my clients enjoy working out at a gym— they're convenient and offer both classes and an opportunity to socialize. However, if you're new to exercise, working out at a gym can be intimidating, especially if you don't know your way around the equipment or you have a lot of weight to lose.

There's a simple solution: Skip the gym and work out at home. You can easily pop in a fitness DVD and get a great workout. You can also burn calories and tone up by walking, hiking, or jogging in the park, on a hiking trail, or around the neighborhood. Remember, exercise should be enjoyable. If gyms aren't your thing, there's no reason to join one.

That said, not liking gym workouts is one thing. Avoiding the gym because you're intimidated is another. If you're in the latter group, I encourage you to take steps to increase your comfort level. You might make a one-time appointment with a personal trainer, who can introduce you to the equipment, design a basic routine for you, and take you through it once. Another thing to consider: You might push yourself harder at a gym. My patients who have transitioned from home exercise to gym workouts push themselves harder at the gym, in front of others, than they do at home.

START SLOW, BUT MOVE DAILY

There's a lot of confusion about how much physical activity we really need. That's because there are different recommendations for health, for maintaining weight, and for losing weight. But all you need to know is that regardless of which goal you're aiming for, you've got to move.

For health, the government recommends 30 minutes of moderate-intensity physical activity five days a week or 75 minutes a week of a vigorous-intensity activity. To both of those recommendations, add two days a week of muscle-strengthening activities.

MODERATE VERSUS VIGOROUS INTENSITY

Moderate-Intensity Activity

- You're working hard enough to raise your heart rate.

- You're sweating.

- You can talk, but not sing the words to your favorite song.

Examples: brisk walking, riding your bike on level ground, doing water aerobics, playing doubles tennis

Vigorous-Intensity Activity

- You're breathing hard and fast.

- Your heart rate is significantly raised.

- You can't talk without pausing for a breath.

Examples: jogging, swimming laps, riding a bike hard or up hills, playing singles tennis

You can do either type of activity, or a mix of the two each week. Rule of thumb: One minute of vigorous-intensity activity is roughly equal to two minutes of moderate-intensity activity. If you want to exercise at a more vigorous intensity, build up to it. As your fitness level increases, you might swap brisk walking for a slow jog, and then a full run.

Muscle-Strengthening Activities

- Lifting weights

- Working with resistance bands

- Doing exercises that use your body weight for resistance (i.e., push-ups, sit-ups)

- Heavy gardening (i.e., digging, shoveling)

- Yoga

To lose weight, cutting calories is the way to go, says the Institute of Medicine (IOM). Any amount of exercise you do beyond that helps to increase the amount of weight you lose. So the 30 minutes, five days a week "prescription" for health on pages 272–273 is also perfect for weight loss. You'll reduce your risk of diabetes, heart disease, and other chronic diseases, plus burn calories.

Meeting those guidelines isn't as tough as you think. Any activity counts, as long as you do it at a moderate or vigorous intensity for at least 10 minutes at a time.

If you're among the 60 percent of Americans who are completely inactive, use your common sense, please. Don't go from long-term inactivity to running on a treadmill. Start slowly—say, 10 or 15 minutes of brisk walking a day. As you raise your fitness level, push beyond those 30 minutes. Go to 35, then 40, then 45 . . . you get the idea.

It's important to increase the length and/or intensity of your workouts at a pace that feels comfortable. Because when you reach your goal weight, you'll need to continue with this exercise regime to keep those lost pounds lost. While the IOM recommends an hour a day of moderate-intensity exercise for weight-loss maintenance, some of my patients maintain their weight loss with less exercise—not a lot less, but less. I encourage my patients to do some physical activity five days a week for one hour.

Remember, this 60-minute period can actually

be enjoyable! Go sledding with your kids in the winter, swim in the summer, walk, do yoga, play volleyball or even Ping-Pong—it's your choice, as long as you do it at a moderate intensity. And if you also take those extra steps whenever possible, you are ahead of the game.

If you have diabetes, heart disease, or another chronic condition, don't exercise at all until you talk with your doctor. He or she can help you devise a plan that matches your abilities. Even if you can't do 30 minutes a day, do as much as you can. Any physical activity at all is better than none.

Often, the biggest exercise hurdle for my patients is simply getting started. Once they do, they're happy they did. Of course, there are always the rebels.

I don't have time to exercise! My schedule is crazy.

Small Change Solution: Everyone's schedule is crazy. That's why you write to-do lists or use the calendar software on your phone or computer, right? And that's why you should literally schedule your workout into your day. Make an "appointment" with your favorite fitness DVD, weights at the gym, or yoga class, and chances are you'll keep that appointment.

Also consider when your schedule is least

"crazy"—morning, afternoon, or evening? Schedule your exercise appointments during that time. Before long, your workout will become a regular part of your day.

Another trick that works: Put on your workout clothes, even when you don't want to. Once you make it that far, you're more likely to actually work out. That's what one of my patients, Meredith, twenty-nine, does. She, too, used to blame her unpredictable schedule for why she didn't work out regularly. "Every day, I'd tell myself I would leave the office early and exercise, but something always came up or I was too tired to go," she said.

Then she began to put on her gym clothes immediately when she arrived home from work. "That's the key for me," she said. She's clearly doing something right, because she's maintained her twenty-five-pound weight loss for eight months.

I work all day and come home to household chores and a demanding family life. All my time is spent on my family. There's simply none left for me—or an exercise program.

Small Change Solution: Being a working parent can make it seem virtually impossible to carve out time for yourself. But keep trying. "Me time" makes for a happier you, and a better parent. Besides, your health benefits your entire family.

But let's stay realistic: If you're buried during the week, get your exercise on the weekends. In my view, it's OK to be a "weekend warrior" as long as you're careful not to injure yourself. Have your partner watch the kids while you get a walk in or get to the gym for an hour. If you have a very young child and no one to watch him, plop him in his stroller and go for a brisk walk. It is important for children to see their parents engage in physical activity. Remember, they learn from you.

Small Change Move-Daily Tips

1. Schedule an appointment to exercise. If you don't plan for it, it won't happen.

2. Make sure you're doing the appropriate amount of exercise to either lose or maintain your weight.

3. Bring your exercise gear with you to work so you can either work out during lunch if possible or go right to the gym afterward. If you must go home first, change into your workout clothes immediately.

4. If you exercise at home in the morning, lay your workout clothes by your bed, so you can put them on as soon as you wake up. If you work out at night, place them in the spot that tempts you to get lazy—on the couch, perhaps.

5. If you can't work out during the week, at least do so on the weekends. And once you're successful on weekends, try to add a workout in the middle of the week.

✔ How's It Going?

Are you writing in your food journal every day? Are you recording all nibbles and beverages, including alcohol?

STEP IT UP!

Walking. What's not to love? It can help slim your waistline; strengthen your heart, lungs, and bones; and boost your mood. It's free. It doesn't take an hour out of your already-jammed-up schedule. And you already know how to do it.

The best part of walking: It's customizable. You can take a brisk 30-minute walk before, during, or after work. If you're pressed for time, you can break that half hour into three 10-minute power walks. One study of sedentary women showed that short bouts of brisk walking (three 10-minute walks per day) were as effective in reducing body fat as one 30-minute walk per day. You can even do it on the fly—every extra step you take makes a difference.

Speaking of extra steps, if you're not quite ready to commit to a walking program, consider using a pedometer to spur you to move more and sit less. Clipped to your belt, a pedometer senses the motion of your body, counts your footsteps, and converts that count into distance by using the length of your stride. And there's something about a pedometer that spurs you to take just one more step . . . and then another.

For such a small gadget, a pedometer can produce big results. Studies have shown that taking 10,000 steps a day—which equates to roughly five miles—can promote weight loss and benefit blood pressure and heart health. Although 10,000 steps sounds like a lot, amassing them is easier than it sounds. Throughout your day, you have ample opportunities to make your 10,000-step goal. *Look* for opportunities to be active! At the airport, don't take the moving walkway—race to catch your connecting flight. (When my kids were younger, I used to race them.) On those long escalators at the mall or subway stations don't be one of the people who stand on the right. "Pass" those standers on the left!

Pick the Perfect Pedometer

Perfect for you, of course. While all pedometers count steps, they use different methods. In general order of accuracy, these methods include a piezoelectric accelerometer, a coiled spring mechanism, and a hairspring mechanism.

Beyond showing your step total and/or calculating distance, you can stay plain or get fancy. The top features include calorie estimates, clocks, stopwatches and speed estimators, and pulse-rate readers (but don't expect too much accuracy on the calorie estimates). Most department stores, including Walmart and Target, sell pedometers. So do sporting good stores. You can also buy a pedometer online, on sites such as Amazon and eBay. And even some cellphones today come with a pedometer.

Whether you want a basic pedometer or one with all the bells and whistles, keep the following in mind:

- A decent pedometer shouldn't set you back more than $20 or so, but the expensive models may have features

---

that appeal to you. For example, if you're a technophile, you might like a pedometer that uploads your walking data and creates graphs and charts of your activity. Some brands work as a pedometer only, while others use foot pods or GPS sensors to more accurately gauge speed or distance.

- However, avoid pedometers that are given away as promotions. They tend to be cheaply made and inaccurate.

- A pedometer should be comfortable to wear all day and be held securely by its clip.

- The display should be easy to read without removing the unit from your waistband, and protected so that bumps don't punch a button and reset the count. (A protective cover prevents accidental resetting.)

- You should be able to move from function to function easily.

- Don't forget batteries!

As you might guess, I take my own advice—my husband and kids know that when they're with me, I'm taking the stairs and hoping they join me! But even though putting one foot in front of the other is the easiest form of exercise there is, I still hear excuses.

I have no time to walk!

Small Change Solution: Come on. Millions of Americans walk for weight control and health, and most of them have jobs, kids, and lives. The difference between you and these willing walkers: They've discovered that when it comes to exercise, you don't "make time." You take it.

While you have to be ready to make that commitment, you have to start somewhere. How about weekend walks? You might consider walking in the morning, before weekend chores and errands, and inviting your husband and kids to join you. You'll all get some exercise (it's important to model healthy behavior for your kids) and have a chance to bond as a family after a hectic week. If you have a dog, take him for long walks instead of short ones; he (or she) also needs exercise and it will make for a happier pet. Single? Invite a friend— you can support and motivate each other, and maybe even meet other single walkers. After a few weeks, you may surprise yourself and branch out to lunchtime walks, and then walks before or after work.

I'm exhausted just thinking about taking 10,000 steps in a day! There's no way I could do it.

Small Change Solution: Sure you can, because you don't have to *start* with 10,000 steps. To begin, count your average daily steps for one week. Clip on your pedometer every morning and wear it until bedtime. Record your daily steps in your journal. By week's end, you'll know how many steps you take a day, on average.

Once you've got your baseline, increase your daily steps by 500 each week, until you're at 10,000 a day. For example, if your week of tracking shows you currently average 3,000 steps a day, aim for 3,500 steps a day in week two, 4,000 steps a day in week three, and so on. In fourteen weeks, you should reach 10,000 steps, no sweat.

Small Change Step-It-Up Tips

1. During your lunch break, go for a walk instead of just sitting at your desk.

2. Take the stairs instead of the escalator or elevator.

3. Take an activity break—walk to a coworker's office instead of sending them an e-mail, or get up and walk around your home when you make or take a call on your phone.

4. Park your car a little farther away from your destination.

5. Get out of the bus/subway a stop earlier and walk the extra distance.

FIND YOUR MOTIVATION

There are many good reasons to exercise. But to stick to an exercise routine day in and day out, you need more than good reasons. You need a *mission*—one powerful reason to get your butt off the couch when that little voice inside says, "I don't wanna."

When you find that reason, you will find your motivation. But you need to seek motivation. Above all, you need to make it *personal*.

One of my motivations is my yoga community. Besides my true love of the practice, I really do enjoy practicing with my friends. Sometimes when I wake up in the morning and feel lazy, I think of my friends and teacher who await me—and I'm out the door.

Maybe your motivation is some*one*—your partner, a friend, a coworker, or another family member. You can join a gym together or simply walk together every day. Remember, as they're motivating you to pull on your sweats and get active, you're helping them! As you inspire and motivate each other, you both benefit.

Perhaps there's a cause that's dear to your heart. If so, run, walk, or cycle to help it raise money. And it's not a onetime deal because you can train for it. There are so many causes to choose from: breast cancer, diabetes, the local animal shelter, an organization that helps battered women or the homeless. Each step you take, each mile you cycle, you're doing good and being active in the process.

If you're really short on inspiration, a personal trainer may be the answer. An hour a week of one-on-one with a can-do, motivational trainer who knows his or her stuff can make you want to stay active the rest of the week. And because they believe you can do it, you begin to believe it, too.

Once my patients find "their" motivation, they enjoy being active. But sometimes there can be stumbling blocks along the way.

Every time I start an exercise plan, I drop it within two weeks. Nothing seems to motivate me!

Small Change Solution: Maybe you need constant reminders of just why you want to get active. Have you ever tried creating a "motivation list"? It's simple, but it can really get you moving when you can't think of a single reason you should.

On a piece of paper, write down every good thing that will happen if you get your butt off the couch and go for your 30-minute walk or to your yoga class. Here are some examples:

- You'll have more energy for your family at night.

- You'll be able to fit into every single piece of clothing you own and then decide whether or not you want to buy new items.

- You'll live a longer, healthier life, which enables you to achieve your dreams (to walk the Appalachian Trail, or simply to enjoy time with your grandchildren).

- You'll be less self-conscious in a bathing suit in public.

Those are some examples; yours may be very different, so give it some serious thought. When you've completed your list, keep it someplace handy, on the refrigerator, at your desk, or even in your wallet. The next time you need an extra shot of motivation, go grab your list. There are your motivations, right there in your hand!

I'm just too tired to exercise.

Small Change Solution: I know you feel tired. I know you think you're too tired. But actually, you're tired because you're not active. Even normally active people who skip a week of workouts begin to feel sluggish, lethargic, and unmotivated. So no matter how sluggish you feel, push yourself for the first week or two. I guarantee that your fatigue will be replaced with energy.

One thing that can help: Work out at the time of day that you're most energized and alert. Morning is always the best time for me and most of my patients—the longer in the day you wait to exercise, the more excuses you will develop not to go. But if you're not a morning person, or your schedule won't permit it, during your lunch hour or after work is fine. The key, obviously, is to make it happen.

Small Change Get-Inspired Tips

1. Find your exercise "why." Make a motivation list.

2. To inspire yourself, inspire someone else. Find an exercise buddy.

3. Make being active count. Get involved with a cause.

4. If you can't get motivated yourself, get help from a personal trainer.

5. Work out early in the day, if possible.

FIDGET TO FIGHT FAT

Tap your toes. Drum your fingers. Cross and uncross your legs. Pace the room as you brainstorm. In a word, fidget like a third-grader on the last day of school—you'll burn calories. The scientific term for fidgeting—nonexercise activity thermogenesis (NEAT for short)—was coined in a study conducted at the Mayo Clinic, which concluded that someone who fidgets can burn up to 350 calories more a day than someone who is stationary.

While NEAT isn't a replacement for exercise, it does burn extra calories. And when you're trying to lose weight, every calorie helps.

ARE YOU READY TO MOVE ON?

This Small Change is a big deal. While it's probably the most challenging to implement, it's also the one that can make the most difference—not just in your weight, but in your mood and attitude. It's a great day when you head to the gym, or set off on your walk, and you realize that you're actually looking forward to it! Are you there yet? Take the final Small Change Success Test.

Small Change Success Test

1. Have you turned being active into "playtime" instead of drudgery?

2. Did you begin to get active slowly, and are you getting 30 minutes of exercise a day?

3. Are you looking for opportunities to walk more during the day?

4. Have you found your primary reason to stay active?

If you answered yes to no more than two of the items above, give yourself a break—and more time. Committing to a regular exercise routine isn't the easiest thing to do. But if you strive to make your workout play, before long you'll be looking forward to that time of day—and your health, and weight, will show it!

If you've answered yes to at least three questions, congratulations. If you've read the book from cover to cover and made the Small Changes in order, you don't need my congratulations. You're no doubt receiving them from others!

Nice work. Now, there's just one thing left to learn: to keep those hard-won results for the rest of your life.

CONCLUSION

▼▲▼▲▼▲▼▲▼▲▼

Weight Loss for Life

Congratulations! No matter which Small Change you began your journey with, you've reached the end of this book, and the beginning of a very different journey: maintaining your weight and new healthy lifestyle. But before we go on, take a moment to give yourself a hand. Making lifestyle changes is never easy, but the benefits, as I think you have discovered, are worth it.

Now I hope you're up for a new challenge, because on the day you meet your weight loss goal—whether you've already done so or have a ways to go—the easiest part of your journey is actually over, and the hard part begins: keeping the weight off. There's no way around it: To maintain your new, healthier weight, you have to want it—and work for it, continuously.

However, the work isn't as hard as you might think. My Small Changes were designed to become a part of your everyday life—a part of *you*. Hopefully, by now, at least a few of them have become as automatic as brushing your teeth. While not every Small Change will be easy, some will be easier than others. Focus on those, and keep working to add more of them to your life. The more of them you can integrate into your life, the easier you'll find it to keep those lost pounds lost.

Will you do each Small Change perfectly, all the time? Nope. But what matters is that you stick to as many of them as you can, a day at a time. When you do that, you're moving in the right direction and all those changes will show up in the mirror and with your health. Take it one Small Change at a time—no need to rush things—and be proud of what you *have* accomplished so far.

Two of my patients, Patricia and Hank, have been seeing me together for the past four years. While I'd love to tell you that they've made all ten Small Changes and reached their goal weights, I can't. What I *can* tell you, however, is that they're both thinner than they were four years ago—Patricia by fourteen pounds, and Hank by seven. Hank, who is at risk for type 2 diabetes, is still healthy. And while they haven't yet tackled every Small Change, they've mastered quite a few. Their dinners always include salads, they eat more fruits, veggies, and fish, and they don't *always* overindulge on a special occasion. When they're ready, they'll make all the changes, and while I'm hard on them, I admire their resilience. They take their slips in stride and strive to do better than they did the day before—and that determination is what keeps them in the game. So you see, perfection isn't the goal; perseverance is. And if they can persevere, one day at a time, so can you!

THE "10 COMMANDMENTS" OF WEIGHT LOSS FOR LIFE

Each mastered Small Change brings you closer to your goal: a longer, healthier life. But the changes don't just help you lose weight—they help you keep it off for good. Let's recap.

Small Change 1: Create a healthy eating schedule. Don't skip meals. Eat breakfast, lunch, dinner, and ideally two snacks a day. When you eat every three to four hours, you're less likely to overindulge or eat the wrong foods.

Small Change 2: Brighten your plate, naturally. Build all your meals with low-calorie fruits and veggies. They help fill you up without filling you out. Half your plate should contain veggies, especially at dinner. Have fruit for dessert more often than not.

Small Change 3: Think before you drink (sip, guzzle, or chug). Always think about your drink. Don't waste calories on sugary beverages with no nutritional content. Choose water, seltzer, low-fat milk, and other low-calorie, sugar-free beverages instead.

Small Change 4: Give your carbs a makeover. Carbs are not the enemy. What really matters is how much, what kind, and which "extras." Choose high-fiber carbs, watch those portions, and dress them with low-calorie and low-fat toppings.

Small Change 5: Go easy on the "extras" and make savory swaps for old standbys. Most important words to learn: *on the side.* Swap high-fat dressings and toppings for low-fat alternatives, whether you're eating in or dining out.

Small Change 6: Skinny your meat. Eat less high-fat beef, more fish, and remove skin from poultry. Bypass fried meats, chicken, and fish for those that are grilled, broiled, and roasted. Be adventurous and have one meatless meal per week.

Small Change 7: Eat the right kinds (and amounts) of fat. Eating fat doesn't make you fat, but eating too much of it will. Incorporate healthy fats into your meals—for example, an ounce of nuts, a fifth of an avocado, and a teaspoon of healthy oils (olive, canola, omega-3s). Limit the amount of processed foods you eat.

Small Change 8: Tame your sweet tooth and your saltshaker. Start your day with a balanced breakfast and have healthy snacks on hand at all times, and you'll help keep your cravings at bay.

Small Change 9: Share food and good times with advance planning—and without guilt. Don't use vacations, holidays, and other events as an excuse to overeat. Make special occasions more about socializing and less about the food. Always have an eating plan in place before an event.

Small Change 10: Get moving. You need to make the time. Devote 30 minutes, five days a week to a brisk walk or other workout, walk more in your everyday life, and strive to make workout time, playtime. Above all, never lose sight of your exercise "why"—when it comes to exercise, motivation is everything!

IF YOU SLIP, PICK YOURSELF UP—ASAP

Of course, we're human, and therefore imperfect, and at times we will overindulge. Even I still eat French fries, pizza, and bagels and drink martinis. I'm okay with that. I don't have to eat perfectly all the time, and neither do you. Eat well 80 percent of the time, and you'll be fine.

Continue to weigh yourself each week. If you gain a pound or two, no worries—that can be water weight. But if you gain more than two pounds, it's time to deal.

If you find yourself slipping, you don't have to stay on the floor. Here's a simple plan to get you on your feet again.

1. Pick up this book and choose the Small Change that's giving you trouble. Then start working the plan that corresponds to that Small Change. Remember, these are small, simple changes, so you needn't change your diet all at once. Just focus on one Small Change at a time, as you did when you began.

2. If you've stopped using your food journal, pick it up again. Record your daily food intake—every bite, sip, and nibble—until you feel that you're back on track.

3. One of the most important things you can do for weight maintenance is to continue to exercise 30 minutes a day, five days a week. Brisk walking and other activities of moderate intensity are fine. It's important to be more active in your daily life, too—take every extra step you can.

Remember the folks in the National Weight Control Registry? They've lost an average of sixty-six pounds and kept off their weight for an average of 5.5 years. Here are some of the weight-control strategies adopted by the majority of them:

- They eat a breakfast every morning (78 percent).
- They step on the scale at least once a week (75 percent).
- They watch less than ten hours of TV a week (62 percent).
- They are active about an hour a day (90 percent). Their favorite activity? Walking.
- They follow a low-fat diet, averaging about 24 percent of their daily calories from fat, and opt for healthy carbs more often than not.

While all *you* have to do is use the Small Changes, these folks' strategies are solid, and their success, inspiring. Just goes to show you that you *can* keep the weight off if you are committed to it!

GO FORWARD AND MAINTAIN

Weight loss is about hitting a number, achieving a goal, and most important, maintaining it. It is about a healthier, more active you who no longer keeps a few pairs of pants in your closet a couple of sizes larger for "just in case."

Christina, fifty-three, has been a patient of mine for three years, and for a few years now has kept off the fifteen pounds she needed to lose. "There are a few dietary rules that have helped me both lose the weight and, more important, maintain it over the last few years," she said. "No more than one serving of red meat per week, at least two servings of fish or shellfish a week, and fruit at least once a day. But the big one for me is portion control, particularly for favorite foods like pasta, pizza, and potatoes. Limiting the portions of those foods has helped tremendously and significantly reduced my cravings for them."

Achieving your goal weight, as Christina has, is satisfying. You have a mission, and when you hit that number, you've accomplished it. Maintenance doesn't necessarily have that kind of satisfying conclusion; it never ends. So where's the reward in that?

Well, to start with, maybe fitting into clothes you always dreamed of wearing. Feeling just fine about bathing-suit season. Getting the results of a cholesterol test from your doctor's office that is normal. Being able to walk up a few flights of stairs without gasping for air, or to run with your children or grandchildren. Showing off the new you at your high school reunion. The list is endless, but everything on it matters—to you and to those who love and care for you.

So there are many rewards, and they all circle back to taking care of you. Taking care of your healthier body. Believing you're worth the effort. Feeling some small measure of satisfaction each time you finish your walk, leave the gym, or enjoy yet another healthy, delicious meal. You'll soon see that rewards keep coming in *all* areas of your life. Following the Small Changes keeps you moving forward.

Once you hit that number on the scale, search for a new motivation to keep you there. Resolve to enjoy the new you. Learn to look for new challenges, new inspirations, and to use them to push yourself further—not to lose more weight, necessarily, but to appreciate and enjoy your accomplishment.

Get ready to take your next journey—and keep up the great work!

APPENDIX

▼▲▼▲▼▲▼▲▼

Burn, Baby, Burn!

There are countless ways to "exercise." The chart below calculates the approximate calories burned during exercises and activities, based on different body weights, for one hour.* If you weigh more, you'll burn more calories. If you weigh less, you'll burn a little less. And the more vigorously you work, the more calories you'll burn.

| Exercise or activity (60 minutes) | Calories burned per | | |
	130 pounds	155 pounds	190 pounds
Aerobics, general	354	422	518
Aerobics, low impact	295	352	431
Backpacking, general	413	493	604
Badminton, social, general	266	317	388
Basketball, game	472	563	690
Bicycling, <10 mph, leisure	236	281	345

* Figures from Wisconsin Department of Health and Family Services.

Exercise or activity (60 minutes)	Calories burned per		
	130 pounds	155 pounds	190 pounds
Bicycling, 10–12 mph, light effort	354	422	518
Bicycling, 12–14 mph, moderate effort	472	563	690
Bicycling, 14–16 mph, vigorous effort	590	704	863
Bicycling, mountain	502	598	733
Bicycling, stationary, general	295	352	431
Bicycling, stationary, vigorous effort	620	739	906
Bowling	177	211	259
Calisthenics, vigorous effort	472	563	690
Calisthenics, light/moderate effort	266	317	388
Canoeing, rowing, light effort	177	211	259
Canoeing, rowing, moderate effort	413	493	604
Circuit training, general	472	563	690
Cleaning, house, general	207	246	302
Croquet	148	176	216
Dancing, aerobic, ballet or modern	354	422	518
Dancing, ballroom, fast	325	387	474
Dancing, ballroom, slow	177	211	259
Dancing, general	266	317	388
Darts, wall or lawn	148	176	216
Fencing	354	422	518
Fishing from boat, sitting	148	176	216
Fishing, general	236	281	345
Football or baseball, playing catch	148	176	216
Football, touch, flag, general	472	563	690
Frisbee playing, general	177	211	259
Gardening, general	295	352	431
Golf, carrying clubs	325	387	474
Golf, general	236	281	345

Exercise or activity (60 minutes)	Calories burned per		
	130 pounds	155 pounds	190 pounds
Golf, miniature or driving range	177	211	259
Golf, pulling clubs	295	352	431
Golf, using power cart	207	246	302
Handball, general	708	844	1035
Health club exercise, general	325	387	474
Hiking, cross-country	354	422	518
Hockey, field	472	563	690
Hockey, ice	472	563	690
Horseback riding, general	236	281	345
Horseback riding, walking	148	176	216
Jogging, general	413	493	604
Judo, karate, kickboxing, tae kwon do	590	704	863
Kayaking	295	352	431
Kickball	413	493	604
Lacrosse	472	563	690
Mowing lawn, general	325	387	474
Mowing lawn, riding mower	148	176	216
Paddleboat	236	281	345
Painting, papering, scraping	266	317	388
Pushing or pulling stroller with child	148	176	216
Race walking	384	457	561
Racquetball, casual, general	413	493	604
Raking lawn	236	281	345
Rock climbing, ascending rock	649	774	949
Rock climbing, rapelling	472	563	690
Rope jumping, fast	708	844	1035
Rope jumping, moderate, general	590	704	863
Rowing, stationary, light effort	561	669	819
Running, general	472	563	690
Running, stairs, up	885	1056	1294
Sailing, boat/board, windsurfing	177	211	259

Exercise or activity (60 minutes)	Calories burned per		
	130 pounds	155 pounds	190 pounds
Shoveling snow, by hand	354	422	518
Shuffleboard, lawn bowling	177	211	259
Skateboarding	295	352	431
Skating, ice, general	413	493	604
Skating, roller	413	493	604
Skiing, cross-country, moderate effort	472	563	690
Skiing, cross-country, light effort	413	493	604
Skiing, cross-country, vigorous effort	531	633	776
Skiing, snow, general	413	493	604
Skiing, water	354	422	518
Skin diving, scuba diving, general	413	493	604
Sledding, tobogganing	413	493	604
Snorkeling	295	352	431
Snow shoeing	472	563	690
Soccer, casual, general	413	493	604
Softball or baseball, fast or slow pitch	295	352	431
Squash	708	844	1035
Stair-treadmill ergometer, general	354	422	518
Stretching, hatha yoga	236	281	345
Surfing, body or board	177	211	259
Swimming laps, freestyle, vigorous effort	590	704	863
Swimming laps, freestyle, moderate effort	472	563	690
Swimming, backstroke, general	472	563	690
Swimming, breaststroke, general	590	704	863
Swimming, leisurely, general	354	422	518
Table tennis, Ping-Pong	236	281	345
Tai chi	236	281	345
Teaching aerobics class	354	422	518

Exercise or activity (60 minutes)	Calories burned per		
	130 pounds	155 pounds	190 pounds
Tennis, general	413	493	604
Tennis, singles	472	563	690
Volleyball, beach	472	563	690
Volleyball, noncompetitive team	177	211	259
Walking, 3.0 mph, mod. pace	207	246	302
Walking, 3.5 mph, uphill	354	422	518
Walking, 4.0 mph, very brisk pace	236	281	345
Water aerobics, water calisthenics	236	281	345
Weight lifting, light or moderate effort	177	211	259
Weight lifting, vigorous effort	354	422	518
Whitewater rafting/kayaking/canoeing	295	352	431

ACKNOWLEDGMENTS
▼▲▼▲▼▲▼▲▼▲▼

First and foremost, I must thank each and every one of my patients, both past and present, because without all of you there would be nothing to write about. And especially for those of you who have a zillion excuses for me every time we meet.

My agent, Celeste Fine, Literary Folio Management, who believed I should have a book from the moment we first spoke. Without her there would be no *Small Change Diet*; she is truly unbelievable.

Julia VanTine Reichart, who started to sound like me before I even said anything. And who kept reminding me that not everyone lives in New York City.

My dear friend Ann Benjamin who has been my personal cheerleader since the day I met her and shared a room on a yoga retreat in Belize.

My favorite yoga yenta, Sherri Rifkin, who introduced me to her world of publishing sitting on our bench in East Hampton drinking our iced coffees (unsweetened, of course).

My mother, Carol Gans, who gave me fresh-squeezed orange juice and natural peanut butter long before I could appreciate them or even like them. And who taught me that hard work does pay off.

My father, Murray Gans, who I am sure must be beaming from above. He would be so.happy that I chose not to be an attorney.

My husband, Bartley Labiner, who never understands why I do half the things I do, especially write a book, but still can't help loving me with all his heart.

And lastly, to my four-legged son, Henry, who sits in my office with my patients all day long and never gets bored with hearing me say the same things over and over again.